7 STEPS TO A PAIN-FREE LIFE

Also by Robin McKenzie

Treat Your Own Back

Treat Your Own Neck

The Cervical and Thoracic Spine: Mechanical Diagnosis and Therapy

The Lumbar Spine: Mechanical Diagnosis and Therapy

The Human Extremities: Mechanical Diagnosis and Therapy

Treat Your Own Shoulder

Treat Your Own Knee

*Against the Tide: Back Pain Treatment—
the Breakthrough: An Autobiography*

7 STEPS TO A PAIN-FREE LIFE

HOW TO RAPIDLY RELIEVE BACK, NECK, AND SHOULDER PAIN

Robin McKenzie

with Craig Kubey

A PLUME BOOK

PLUME
Published by the Penguin Group
Penguin Group (USA) LLC
375 Hudson Street
New York, New York 10014

USA | Canada | UK | Ireland | Australia | New Zealand | India | South Africa | China
penguin.com
A Penguin Random House Company

First published in the United States of America by Dutton,
a member of Penguin Group (USA) Inc., 2000
First Plume printing 2001
First Plume printing (updated edition) 2014

 REGISTERED TRADEMARK—MARCA REGISTRADA

ISBN 978-0-14-218069-3

Printed in the United States of America
10 9 8 7 6 5 4 3 2 1

Set in Warnock Pro with DIN Next
Designed by Daniel Lagin

To my wife, Joy

CONTENTS

Preface: The Chance Discovery   ix

Acknowledgments   xiii

Introduction to the First Edition by Craig Kubey   xvii

Introduction to the Second Edition by Craig Kubey   xxiii

Chapter 1. You Can Stop Back and Neck Pain   1

Chapter 2. How Your Back and Neck Work and Why They Hurt   9

Chapter 3. Back Problems   18

Chapter 4. Common Causes of Lower Back Pain   26

Chapter 5. The McKenzie Method Exercises for the Back   55

Chapter 6. When to Do the Back Exercises   78

Chapter 7. Instructions for People with Acute Lower Back Pain   90

Chapter 8. Special Back Situations   95

Chapter 9. Common Back Remedies and Solutions   107

Chapter 10. Neck Problems   111

Chapter 11. Common Causes of Neck Pain   124

Chapter 12. The McKenzie Method Exercises for the Neck   138

Chapter 13. When to Do the Neck Exercises   158

Chapter 14. Instructions for People with Acute Neck Pain   163

Chapter 15. Panic Pages for the Back   166

Chapter 16. Panic Pages for the Neck   169

Chapter 17. Shoulder Problems   172

Chapter 18. The Shoulder and Neck Region   183

Chapter 19. Common Causes of Shoulder Pain   190

Chapter 20. The McKenzie Method for the Shoulder   209

Chapter 21. The McKenzie Method Exercises for the Shoulder   212

Chapter 22. When to Do the Shoulder Exercises   222

Appendix A: How to Find a McKenzie-Trained
Health Care Practitioner   231

Appendix B: Products for the Back and Neck   235

About the Author, Collaborator, and Coauthors   237

Index   241

PREFACE
THE CHANCE DISCOVERY

I PRACTICE PHYSIOTHERAPY IN NEW ZEALAND. IN THE DIFFERENT
English spoken in the United States, this means I am a physical therapist. In 1956, I was only a few years into my career when a "Mr. Smith" came into the office. He complained of pain that extended from the right side of his lower back to his right knee. It was difficult for him to stand upright. He could bend forward, but he could not bend backward. For three weeks I treated him with heat and ultrasound. These were well-accepted therapeutic techniques then and remain so now. Nevertheless, Mr. Smith did not improve at all.

Then, late on a Wednesday, Mr. Smith came in for another appointment. I greeted him and said, "Go into that treatment room, please. Undress and then lie facedown on the table, and I'll be in to see you."

Mr. Smith complied—to the letter. I didn't know it, but another physiotherapist had left the therapy table at an odd angle: the front was elevated 45 degrees. Mr. Smith lay facedown on that table, his pelvis and legs horizontal, his torso sharply elevated in a position called *extension*.

But I got a phone call, and then another physiotherapist needed to consult me. And so five minutes passed before I could attend to Mr. Smith. I knocked on his door, walked briskly in, and then froze. To my horror, I saw Mr. Smith lying in the bizarre position just described. Not only was the position odd; in 1956 the position was considered by the medical profession to be one that would cause damage to most any patient. I thought, "My God! What has he done? Has he made his injury much worse?"

"How are you doing, Mr. Smith?" I asked gingerly.

"It's the best I've been," he replied in sunny tones. "All the pain in the leg is gone."

I was astounded and mightily relieved, but I wanted to know more. "How's the low back?" I inquired.

"The funny thing is, the pain is a little worse, but it's moved from the right side over to the center."

"How are you tolerating that pain?"

"Better. It's better when it's in the middle there."

Then he stood up.

He could do this without pain!

I asked him to try carefully to bend forward and backward. As you will recall, previously he could bend forward but not backward.

Now, after those five minutes in that strange position, he suddenly could bend backward with only minor pain.

His standing up did nothing to reverse the gains he had experienced on the table: there still was no pain in his leg, and the back pain remained centralized.

I began to recover my equilibrium. "Oh, yes, that's fine," I said, stumbling only a little. But I wanted to be sure no damage had been done. "Could you walk around a bit?" I asked him.

Mr. Smith walked around the treatment room. He walked quite normally. I was relieved. I felt that he had improved so much that we could ask for nothing more that day.

"Well, that's long enough for today," I said. "Come back tomorrow and we'll try it again."

The next day, Mr. Smith was back. And we repeated the same "treatment." After Mr. Smith had maintained that odd position on the table for about five minutes, all his remaining symptoms were gone.

Mr. Smith taught me about extension. Learning from his remarkable recovery, I was able to develop exercises and postural-correction techniques involving extension and, later, flexion. On the following pages I will explain all these to you. Thanks to Mr. Smith, you are probably just one book away from being well on the road to recovery.

IMPORTANT: If you have severe back or neck pain or are having your first episode of back or neck pain, do not use this book. See a physician or other health care provider.

If you are now suffering from acute lower back pain, and have previously consulted a health care provider about your back pain, skip to Chapter 7, "Instructions for People with Acute Lower Back Pain."

Similarly, if you have acute neck pain *right now*, and have previously consulted a health care provider about your neck pain, skip to Chapter 14, "Instructions for People with Acute Neck Pain."

If you have back or neck pain that troubles you but is not acute, start with Chapter 1.

ACKNOWLEDGMENTS

ROBIN MCKENZIE

To my patients who entrusted me with their care over the past forty years, I give my thanks and gratitude for teaching me all I know. I pass this on to you, the reader, and trust that you too can benefit.

CRAIG KUBEY

I am grateful to the many McKenzie-affiliated health practitioners in the United States who generously provided advice and other assistance in connection with this book. They include Dave Pleva, Vert Mooney, M.D., Ron Donelson, M.D., and McKenzie-credentialed physical therapists Todd Edelson, Gudrun Morgan, Aidan O'Connor, Mary Sheid, Gerald Stern, Mary Stern, and Mark Werneke. Thanks also to Stacey Lyon of the McKenzie Institute U.S.A., who helped to put me in touch with the preceding physical therapists. I also thank Alan Kubey for computer assistance and Karen Kubey for photography; I thank them as well as Maki Kubey and Elizabeth Kubey for putting up with my work on this book.

ALL OF US

We thank our literary agency, RLR Associates (Scott Gould, Jonathan Diamond, Lisa Dicker, Jennifer Unter, Manuela Barbuiani, Gretchen Topping, Jason White, et al.), for its diligent work on this project. Further, we express our appreciation to the editorial, production, and publicity people at Dutton (beginning with editor in chief Brian Tart; his assistant, Kara Howland; and copyeditor John Paine) for their extensive efforts to meet the extraordinary demands of the project that produced this book. At Plume, we'd like to thank the publisher of this new, dramatically expanded edition, editor in chief Phil Budnick, as well as Matthew Daddona, Jaya Miceli, Clare Ferraro, Norina Frabotta, and Katie Hurley. We also thank Jan McKenzie, former general manager of Spinal Publications New Zealand Ltd, who handled the New Zealand administrative side of producing the original edition with extraordinary intellect, effort, diligence, diplomacy, and humor. For this new edition, we thank Rachel Mason, Jan's successor as general manager, who was enormously smart, quick, and helpful. We further acknowledge the precise and thorough work of previous general manager Jenny Bertelsen.

And we must mention our other friends in New Zealand:

We thank Stephen May, Rob Hughes, Ezequiel Gherscovici, Kate Allison, Carole Sweney, Rowley Watson, and Sue Lord for assistance with early work on the shoulder section. Regarding photographs in the book, we also thank our models Helen Macdonald, Brian McLean, and Gorman Ngai.

Further, we acknowledge the creative expertise and guidance provided by Rachel Mason at Spinal Publications (already thanked earlier in another connection).

We also thank Caroline Budge, Daniel Allean, Jono Smith, and istockphoto.com.

Finally, we acknowledge the thousands of patients of Robin McKenzie and his associates who unknowingly provided most of the resolutions for back, neck, and shoulder pain that are described in this book.

DEDICATIONS

Robin McKenzie's dedication appears on page v. Craig Kubey dedicates this book to his wife, Maki.

INTRODUCTION TO
THE FIRST EDITION

INTRODUCTIONS TO IMPORTANT BOOKS ARE USUALLY WRITTEN BY experts or celebrities. Or, even better, by experts who *are* celebrities. But I am neither an expert nor a celebrity. I am an attorney who gave up a public service legal career to become a writer. But most important to you, the reader, I am a beneficiary of the McKenzie Method. And I want you to be a beneficiary too.

As you read these words, it is likely (because you chose to pick up this book) that you have back pain or neck pain. I've been there. The main reason I'm not there right now is Robin McKenzie.

I have had plenty of good luck in my life and plenty of bad, but I have had the astonishingly bad luck to get not just one whiplash injury caused by a rear-end auto collision, but three. I have also had the more common experience of developing lower back pain during my forties.

Because there are more back patients than neck patients, let's start with the back. For years I had occasional minor, very tolerable lower back pain for no reason known to me. But I'm a runner: track and cross-country in high school, track at the University of California, Berkeley. One day on a family trip to Santa Cruz, California, I went for a short run in some rolling hills. No back pain during the run.

But when I stopped, I had back pain that was *severe*. My family was a mile away, and it was a painful struggle to walk back to them. Back home, the pain was even worse. I remember one day when my wife and I were downtown and the car was a half block away. I asked her to go to the car and pick me up: the back pain was bad enough that I didn't even want to walk that half block.

But having already benefited from the McKenzie exercises for the neck, I read the McKenzie exercises for the back. I focused on Back Exercise 3, Extension in Lying. Immediately, the back pain was better. In a few days it was so minor that it was of no concern to me.

I also learned that I was wrong in my analysis of what had happened. People who run without pain but find their backs hurting immediately afterward blame the running. Same thing with other sports. But McKenzie says—and my experience has borne this out—that typically the problem is not the exercise but what one does afterward. My run had been short, but it had been in hills and at a fairly rapid pace. So when I finished, I was out of breath, and I bent over, hands on knees, just as so many runners and other athletes do after so many types of exercise. This was where I made my mistake. Every indication is that if I had maintained a good posture right after the run, the back symptoms never would have arisen.

Now to all those whiplash injuries. The first one occurred in 1976. I was stopped at a stop sign and my car was struck by a big Cadillac. I was a member of an early health maintenance organization, and right after my injury, there was no way that HMO would let me see an orthopedist. I saw my family doctor there, but after several weeks my symptoms hadn't gotten much better. So without asking for a referral, I made an appointment with an orthopedist. He had eight patients an hour, and he spent most of our short time together expressing his astonishment that I had gotten to see him at all.

In search of relief, I eventually saw seven doctors: one primary care physician and six orthopedists. I was treated with heat, ultrasound, hands-on physical therapy, aspirin (this was before ibuprofen), Valium (as a muscle relaxant), and a hard cervical collar followed by a soft cervical collar. All these things helped some, but none helped in any dramatic way. The pain persisted for more than a year and interfered seriously with my work and social life. I think the only thing that really got rid of the persistent neck pain was the passage of time—September 1976 to January 1978. The only McKenzie I knew about then was a guy in my high school class who played the drums in a rock band.

The next rear-end auto collision came in May 1986. While I was waiting to turn left at an intersection, my car was struck by a Ford Taurus. I was in a lot of pain once again. But this time I went to just one primary care physician and one orthopedist, who referred me to a physical therapist. For months this physical therapist and his associate treated me with hands-on therapies. These two seemed to know their business much better than the physical therapist of 1976, and almost every time I left their office, I felt much better, but for only about a day.

But eventually this physical therapist introduced me to the McKenzie exercises. I gave them a try once in a while, maybe one session on one day (you're supposed to do them about every two hours), then again some weeks later (you're supposed to do them every day until your symptoms get better). They provided a little relief, but the physical therapist didn't impress upon me the full value of these exercises or the importance of doing them *religiously*, which is to say, to do them exactly as McKenzie would have you do them, and to stick with them. Nor did he seem to recognize that certain McKenzie exercises are tailored to certain situations (such as one-sided pain, which was what I had). So my treatment remained mostly of the hands-on variety. And the symptoms again took more than a year to fully resolve.

In 1993, I had a serious flare-up of my neck condition. This was caused when, as I parked my car, I ran into a curb at moderate speed. Most people would not have been bothered by this, but because of my previous neck injuries, within fifteen minutes I had sharp pain.

But almost right away I remembered the McKenzie exercises, Neck Exercise 1, Head Retraction in Sitting, in particular. I did this exercise one time. That is, I retracted my head one time and held the position for about three seconds. The neck pain vanished all at once! In three seconds! (Years later I talked with a McKenzie-trained chiropractor, who said, "That's great when that happens, isn't it?" He had seen these instant cures with many patients.)

I'm not saying the McKenzie Method is ordinarily so successful that you can spend three seconds with it and be pain free. Chances are small you will be that lucky. But once in a while it's just that powerful. And often the first session of exercises provides relief that, while not complete, is quite noticeable.

Auto collision whiplash number three happened in 1995: a Nissan pickup truck. The pain this time was not generally as severe as in the two other accidents, but it just hung on and hung on through several doctors and one physical therapist. I tried the McKenzie Neck Exercise 1 a few times, and it helped some, but not enough. The pain went on for more than a year.

Maybe I should have learned my lesson earlier, but I did not learn it until *after* the resolution of this third whiplash.

That 1995 auto accident was the last one. But there were countless flare-ups, generally associated with driving. In particular, if I'd strike a curb while parking, I'd have immediate pain. It usually would persist for about a day.

After one such microcollision, the pain was sharper than usual, and it was on one side. I decided to review the McKenzie exercises more carefully. I skimmed through Neck Exercises 1 through 4 and then came to Exercise 5, Side Bending of the Neck. I realized for the first time that this exercise was for the specific situation I was in: pain mostly or exclusively on one side. My pain was on the right side, probably because the pain from the 1995 accident had been there. It had gone away but left me vulnerable.

I did Exercise 5 a few times, and the pain was dramatically reduced in the very first session. I did it for one or two more sessions the same day, and it was just about gone. Soon it had entirely disappeared.

So my message is this: *don't skim, don't be careless, don't just glance at the exercises and make a "reasonable" attempt.* There is *genius* in these exercises, but you must do them *exactly* as Robin McKenzie says. Read every word of every exercise and figure out which one or ones fit your back pain or your neck pain. Do the exercise or exercises *exactly* as Robin instructs you. Do it as many times as he says in each session. Do it as many times a day as he says to, if your schedule in any way permits that. And do the exercises in the right order. If Robin says to do Exercise 1, then 6, then 1, and then 2, do them in that order! This guy McKenzie has been developing these exercises since 1956, and he knows what he's talking about.

You will know all this in your heart only once you have followed his advice (and mine here). When you find out just how right he is, it's an emotional experience. When the pain suddenly declines or even vanishes, you feel relieved; you feel grateful. You feel like finding out how to reach McKenzie and calling him on the phone. His wisdom is seen not just in the results you get, but in your experience as you do the exercises.

Neck Exercise 2, Neck Extension in Sitting, is a great example of this. Robin says to retract your head, then tilt it back as though looking at the sky, then, with your head tilted, repeatedly turn your nose a half inch from the midline to the right and left, all the while tilting still farther back. It's amazing to find that even though you thought you had tilted your head back all the way, you can tilt it still farther back—but only if you turn your nose a little to the right, then to the left, just as he says.

I have paid the price for not following the McKenzie exercises closely enough. No one—no doctor, no physical therapist—had told me how important it was to do the exercises exactly as Robin McKenzie would have you do them. I've paid the price in years of pain and hundreds of medical and physical therapy appointments, 95 percent of which I now believe were unnecessary and therefore a waste of valuable time, not to mention my insurance company's money and my own (those co-payments).

Despite my emphasis on the exercises, it's important to stress two other facts. One is that although McKenzie is known for "extension"—bending the back or neck to a straight position or past that position—his method is much more than that. Even his exercises in some cases involve flexion, which is the opposite of extension. The other is that a back or neck patient will do best if he or she focuses on more than the exercises. That is, the reader should understand the entire McKenzie Method, which includes not only the exercises but a brief discussion of human anatomy, and which concentrates heavily on correct posture as both a preventive and corrective means of dealing with back and neck pain.

Two additional personal points:

1. When you have back or neck pain, especially neck pain, you may feel that your painful area is too fragile to mess around with. Your instinct may be to use ice, lie down, not risk making the injury worse. If you have a legitimate medical concern here, such as a serious injury, sure, rest, see a doctor, be sure it's safe to do the exercises. If it's your first neck injury, Robin himself says to see a doctor before using the exercises.

But if your injury isn't severe, just painful, try the exercises. You may be amazed to find that you probably aren't so fragile after all. You can tolerate the exercises. You may feel very rapid relief.

2. If you don't feel immediate relief, remember what McKenzie will tell you: sometimes relief doesn't come right away; sometimes the exercises are painful and you are no better after a session or two or a day or two. But stick with them. You will in all likelihood benefit from your patience.

They say converts are the most impassioned believers, and I've been converted from hoping doctors and physical therapists can help me to realizing that with McKenzie's exercises I can help myself. When I have a back or neck injury or a flare-up, no longer do I wait helplessly for someone to schedule me for an appointment: I read the McKenzie exercises and follow them to the letter. You can too. You should too.

Learn the McKenzie Method, learn the exercises, then do them exactly as instructed. You will very likely be completely free of pain in a surprisingly short amount of time. From one back/neck sufferer to another, I want you to know that this book may be the most effective doctor you have ever had.

—Craig Kubey

INTRODUCTION TO
THE SECOND EDITION

WHY IS THERE A SECOND EDITION? TWO REASONS. ONE IS THAT THE original *7 Steps to a Pain-Free Life* has done phenomenally well in the United States and many other countries. Big sales, flattering reviews. For example, the book shot to *number five in the world* on the bestseller list at Amazon.com. The book has displayed tremendous endurance, running up big sales every year since its publication. In addition, Amazon.com named *7 Steps* the *sixth-best health book of the year*.

The other reason for the new edition is that we now have a great deal of new information for the reader. We have updated the back and neck sections of the book. More important, we are dramatically enlarging the book by adding a big new section on self-treatment of the shoulder. This section's six new, detailed chapters increase the size of the book by approximately 50 percent. Robin McKenzie collaborated on every one of the new chapters.

—Craig Kubey

7 STEPS TO A PAIN-FREE LIFE

1 YOU CAN STOP BACK AND NECK PAIN

I DON'T CLAIM TO HAVE SPENT YEARS OF RESEARCH ATTEMPTING TO find a new and more effective means for treating back and neck pain. In a flash, those means found me. At least I had the presence of mind to recognize a powerful new therapy when it presented itself. And so, through the willingness of Mr. Smith to follow his physiotherapist's advice no matter how ridiculous, I discovered the power of extension. My colleagues and I now refer to the experience with Mr. Smith as "the Chance Discovery." With Mr. Smith and other patients, I rapidly realized that extension is often the key to prompt and effective self-treatment of back pain.

Over the span of four decades, I have continuously refined the treatment method and applied it not only to back injury and back pain but to neck injury and neck pain as well as shoulder injury and shoulder pain. Most specifically, I have identified seven powerful exercises for the back and seven more for the neck. The method, which also includes postural correction, has become known as the McKenzie Method. Medical researchers have verified the effectiveness of the method for both diagnosis and treatment. Many research articles, published in professional journals, support the method's techniques.

The main features of the human spine are the vertebrae—small bony structures that are separated and cushioned by the discs. Distortion of the discs—changes in their shape—often causes pain in the back and neck. The exercises I have developed allow the discs to return to their normal shape. The result is that pain disappears.

The exciting thing is that sometimes the pain disappears almost instantly. In some ways, the exercises appeal to the energetic and dedicated: these exercises are for people who want to stop depending 100 percent on others—health professionals—to take care of them. But at the same time, the exercises may also appeal to the lazy.

The exercises are easy to do. Certain important exercises require the reader to hold a position for about two seconds and repeat the exercise five to ten times. Each exercise session will last no longer than sixty seconds from start to finish. In the early stages of the program, exercise sessions should be repeated seven or eight times a day. To remain pain free for life, readers will need to adopt good posture (even that becomes a comfortable thing to do over time) and perform the exercises twice daily—just two minutes out of their day.

THE PROBLEM

Back pain, neck pain, and shoulder pain are serious and big business. They are serious business because they are vexing: many back pain "sufferers" really are suffering a great deal. Their pain is severe, sometimes disabling, often distracting. Sometimes it shoots down their legs (this is called sciatica). Neck pain can in at least one sense be even worse than back pain: being so close to the head, it's a very personal pain. Like a headache, it's hard—if not impossible—to ignore. It too can be disabling. Shoulder pain presents very similar problems.

If you have back pain, neck pain, or shoulder pain, you may have had to stop playing sports. If your back pain is bad enough, you may not even be able to walk. Back, neck, or shoulder pain may have kept you home from work.

It may surprise you to know that back pain and neck pain are related. Most neck sufferers also have or will have back pain, and a large percentage of back sufferers also have or will have neck pain. Due to problems such as poor posture, a man or woman with back pain is more likely to develop neck pain than is a person without back trouble. Some patients suffer from shoulder pain as well as back or neck symptoms.

Despite the magnitude of the problem, most people do not get adequate and cost-effective treatment for their back, neck, or shoulder pain. They continue to suffer month after month, year after year.

Chronic lower back pain is probably the most extensive and costly medical problem in the world. It seems that everyone has back pain. The consensus, based on many scientific studies, is that during their lifetimes more than 80 percent of the people in Western nations suffer at least one episode of back pain severe enough to require bed rest; many others experience back pain that is troubling if not severe. Studies indicate that neck pain presents a severe problem at least once in the lives of 40 percent of the population of these countries. Statistics are not available for shoulder pain, but it can be just as disabling as back or neck pain.

So back, neck, and shoulder pain are *big* business. But how are they *big* business? In just the United States, back pain costs more than $100 billion a year in everything from medical expenses to days lost from work. In 2012, *Money* magazine, citing a study in the *Journal of the American Medical Association*, said the average patient with a bad back spends $6,100 a year on it.

Most people who suffer back and neck pain struggle along on their own. But some visit an orthopedist for an appointment, where the chief beneficiary is the doctor, who may bill $275 for an initial examination. In return for this, the physician often gives the patient nothing more than two prescription slips, one for drugs (which in some cases are ineffective or have unpleasant side effects, or both) and another providing a vague but expensive referral to physical therapy. If drugs and physical therapy don't do the trick, some physicians recommend surgery. There are more than 3.4 million visits for back pain per year to hospital emergency departments.

Sometimes surgery is successful; sometimes it is not. All back and neck surgery is costly and requires a recovery period of several weeks, during which time most patients cannot go to work. Most surgery helps more than it hurts, but some operations reduce only some of a patient's pain, and other surgeries are completely unsuccessful: range of motion is reduced and pain is not.

Physical therapists and chiropractors may bill $150 per appointment for several appointments a week over many consecutive months. The bill can easily mount well into the thousands of dollars. These well-meaning professionals may do little more than briefly reduce pain through what they call *modalities*, but which are nothing more sophisticated or effective than ice, heat, and ultrasound. And who has so much leisure time that he or she can easily find three hours a week for treatment, plus the time it takes to get to and from the therapist?

If you are a typical person suffering back pain, you have recurring pain. The attacks are not getting less frequent; they may even be occurring more often. They may be more disabling than they once were.

Or your problem may not be recurring; rather, it may be bothering you nearly every day, month after month, in which case it is *chronic*. Very likely, it has not responded well to physical therapy, chiropractic care, or medication—whether over-the-counter or prescription.

Or you may have had surgery for your back or neck. Even though you went to a qualified surgeon, the surgery may well have failed to correct your problem.

Every year for thirty-five years I saw a thousand patients. These patients taught me that the only people who really needed my services were those with recurrent or chronic back problems. The rest would get better on their own and stay better for long periods. My thousands of patients also taught me that most of them, and therefore most back and neck patients in general, could learn to manage their own problems once they were taught the right exercises, the exercises I describe in this book.

I even found that despite my best efforts, which conformed to the care given by the best physical therapists in my country and others, I was *getting in the way* of finding out which patients could successfully treat themselves. It became clear that if I used the usual "modalities"—heat, ultrasound, spinal manipulation, or spinal adjustment—and the patient got better, I had at least temporarily eliminated the opportunity to see if exercise was enough.

So it became evident that not only were the exercises a great help to the great majority of patients, but they should be used very early in the treatment of patients. In this way, we could identify the many who could "cure themselves" through exercise at home and the few who did require "hands-on" treatment by a physical therapist or other health practitioner.

Once they were taught self-management, most patients with recurring or chronic problems would willingly shoulder (no pun intended) the responsibility for their own care. Many had lost all hope that they would ever be free of back or neck pain. Many had come to assume that the only relief, even if it was only temporary, would come at the expensive hands of a health care expert. But now they were in charge of their own problem.

They had become used to driving to the office of the physical therapist or chiropractor or physician, waiting to be called into the treatment room, partially undressing, having the health professional "work on them," and driving back to their jobs or homes. These visits, travel included, would take hours every week, and sometimes hundreds of hours a year, that could be put to other use. The patients had become used to seeing large amounts of money transferred to the health professional's office or health maintenance organization— their money or an insurance company's money, or some combination. They had believed they were in a dark, endless tunnel lined with time and money.

Now the patients learned the exercises. They found they were effective. They found they took very little time, a tiny fraction of the time it would take for an appointment. They found they were easy to do. And so they found a light at the end of the tunnel!

Lower back pain affects nearly all of us at some stage of our active adult life. It is therefore one of the most common health problems afflicting mankind. It can follow an event or just accompany aging (and I'm not talking about old age here: many people first encounter recurring or chronic back pain in their thirties, and a sizable number encounter it much earlier). It can be called by many names. Among these are fibrositis, fibromyalgia, slipped disc, degenerative disc disease, arthritis of the lower back, rheumatism, lumbago. When the pain extends into the leg, it is called sciatica.

To most people with lower back pain, the cause of their pain is a mystery. Often it starts without warning and for no obvious reason. It interferes with the most simple activities of living, activities that, until the back pain began, the person took for granted. Activities as simple as walking, sitting, and standing. Less simple activities, such as participating in sports or driving a car or participating in family events, become less pleasant or even unpleasant; often they are avoided. Lower back pain also interferes with the critical "nonactivity" of getting a good night's sleep.

Then, just as unexpectedly, the pain subsides or disappears entirely. When in acute (recent, sharp) pain, we are usually unable to think in a calm, deliberate manner about our trouble. Our mind is focused on getting relief. On the other hand, as soon as we have recovered from an acute episode, most of us quickly forget our lower back problems. (Certainly there are other things to think about, other responsibilities to undertake!)

Therefore, once we have developed recurring back pain, we can do nothing but seek assistance, time and again, to become pain free. Due to a lack of knowledge and understanding, we've been unable to deal with symptoms when they are present, and until now we have had no way of preventing future symptoms.

THE SOLUTION

You can stop your own back, neck, or shoulder pain.

You may have thought that your options were limited to these six:

1. Going to a doctor
2. Going to a physical therapist
3. Going to a chiropractor
4. Using prescription or over-the-counter drugs
5. Some combination of the above
6. Doing nothing and hoping the pain will just go away

In fact, there is a powerful seventh alternative: *you can take care of yourself.* Through simple exercises I explain in this book, you can eliminate—or at least dramatically reduce—your back, neck, or shoulder pain in a matter of minutes.

Mr. Smith gave us the discovery of the power of extension. We have built upon it, and now the McKenzie Method is much more than that. In particular, it includes a method of assessing patients for health professionals to use. But even after decades of development, the heart of the McKenzie Method is still extension: bending or pushing the back or neck into a straight position or past it. Extension is the opposite of flexion, the position that most people assume when sitting or standing at work or leisure. Poor posture, in which people are too often in flexion, is the most common cause of back and neck injury.

We have developed wonderfully easy and effective sets of seven exercises for the back, seven for the neck, and six for the shoulder that challenge such mottos as "You get what you pay for" and "No pain, no gain." The exercises are quick and easy to perform. In a session lasting only a few minutes, many will experience great relief. Most people benefit dramatically from performing only one or two of the seven exercises. The full array of exercises provides a range of weapons for attacking pain and stiffness in the back, neck, and shoulder as well as giving people the tools they need to reduce the risk of future episodes.

The other major contribution of the method is this advice to back, neck, and shoulder sufferers: *treat yourself.* The norm in Western nations is that if you have a medical problem, you see a doctor or other health professional. Yet we have found that the great majority of back, neck, and shoulder sufferers can treat themselves successfully without ever walking into a health professional's office. They can treat themselves successfully through the McKenzie exercises.

Fortunately, there has been movement toward the method. In particular, U.S. federal guidelines from the Agency for Health Care Policy and Research (now the Agency for Healthcare Research and Quality) promote movement, minimal bed rest, patient education, and self-responsibility. (S. Bios et al., 1994, "Acute Low Back Problems in Adults: Clinical Practice Guidelines," Quick Reference Guide No. 14, U.S. Department of Health and Human Services, Agency for Health Care Policy and Research, Rockville, MD.)

The causes of most kinds of common lower back problems are quite clear. First I will explain why lower back pain may occur. Then I will suggest how you can avoid it. Or, if you are having lower back pain right now, I will suggest how you may recover from it and what steps you can take if it reappears.

The main point of this book is that the management of your back is *your responsibility.* Of course you can call on people with particular skills—doctors, physical therapists, or chiropractors—for treatment. But in the end, *only you can really help yourself.* That is, only you can help yourself become pain free not only *during* clinical appointments but *without* appointments. Self-treatment of lower back pain is now widely recommended; it will be more effective in the long-term management of your lower back problems than any other form of treatment.

Dozens of books set out to tell you how to care for your own back, so you may wonder why yet another one is now offered. The reason is that this is the first book ever offered in U.S. bookstores that shows you how to *put your back in* if you are unfortunate enough to have *put it out*. In addition, this book shows you what steps you must take to avoid recurrence.

If you have developed lower back pain or neck pain for the first time, consult a health care professional such as your family doctor, a physical therapist who frequently treats back or neck pain, or a chiropractor. Also seek the advice of such a health care professional if there are complications to your lower back pain; for example, if you have constant pain that travels down your leg all the way to your foot, if you have numbness, if you have muscle weakness, or if, in addition to having back pain, you feel unwell. All these circumstances indicate the need to consult a health professional. If you are not sure whether you should consult such a professional, err on the side of protecting yourself and consult one.

The McKenzie Institute International has provided education and training in the McKenzie Method to more than twenty thousand physical therapists, chiropractors, and physicians around the world. In the event that the exercises and other advice in this book fail to give you sufficient relief from your back or neck problem, consult a health practitioner trained in the McKenzie Method. Being intimately familiar with the McKenzie exercises, these professionals are uniquely qualified to determine whether exercises should be enough to provide you with relief or whether more traditional, "hands-on" means are appropriate. (Indeed, in a relatively small minority of cases, the exercises are not enough.) Very often, a one-on-one session with an expert trained in the McKenzie Method will clarify the nature of your problem and the steps you must take to resolve it.

To find a McKenzie-trained health professional in your area, please see Appendix A.

2 HOW YOUR BACK AND NECK WORK AND WHY THEY HURT

THE CULPRIT: BAD POSTURE

By far the most common cause of back pain and neck pain is poor posture. Therefore, back pain often follows these actions:

- Sitting for a long time
- Bending for a long period or over and over—usually at work
- Lifting heavy objects
- Standing
- Lying down in a position of strain

Similarly, neck pain often follows poor posture in activities such as these:

- Sitting for a long period
- Working in a strained position (such as the office worker who often holds a phone in place between the head and shoulder, or the tractor operator who often rotates his head to look behind him)
- Lying down or sleeping with the head in an awkward position

This book will help you maintain good posture and allow you to eliminate the pain and stiffness that come from bad posture.

THE LORDOSIS

Before you begin the exercises, you must understand what bad posture is. And to do that, you must understand the meaning of the word *lordosis*. This term may sound like a disease or an abnormal condition, but in fact it is a natural feature of the lumbar spine in all people.

A lordosis is an inward curve of the spine. The inward curve in the lower back is called the *lumbar lordosis* (Fig. 2.1). This lordosis is found in the small of the back, just above the waistline. Some people refer to it as the "hollow" in the lower back. The smaller inward curve in the neck is called the *cervical lordosis*.

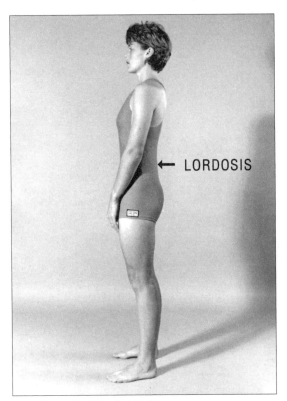

Figure 2.1: Lumbar lordosis

When a person stands upright, the lordosis naturally occurs. Still, the degree of the lordosis varies from person to person and from activity to activity.

Maintenance of the lumbar lordosis isn't just valuable in the effort to make the back healthy and pain free: it is *critical*. Nevertheless, even though the lordosis is natural and despite its importance, it is not always present in all people. In fact, almost everyone loses the lordosis during certain activities, such as bending over and touching one's toes.

The lordosis is lost whenever the lower back is "rounded," as usually occurs when people sit or when they bend forward. And if the lordosis is lost often or for long periods or both, lower back problems frequently result.

ANATOMY

To understand *why* back problems can result from loss of the lordosis, let's quickly focus on human anatomy.

The spine or "backbone" (Fig. 2.2) is made up of vertebrae. Each vertebra looks something like a spool of thread (Fig. 2.3). It is circular and has a hole that runs from top to bottom. There are thirty-three vertebrae: seven in the neck (the *cervical vertebrae*), twelve in the upper back (the *thoracic vertebrae*), five in the lower back (the *lumbar vertebrae*), five fused together in the sacrum (the *sacral vertebrae*), and four rudimentary vertebrae fused together in the coccyx (the *coccygeal vertebrae*; these are the lowest part of the spine and are the vestige of a tail).

With the vertebrae lined up one atop the other, the holes form the spinal canal (Fig. 2.4).

Figure 2.2: The human spine viewed from the side

Figure 2.4: A vertebra

Figure 2.3: The vertebrae are similar to a stack of cotton spools.

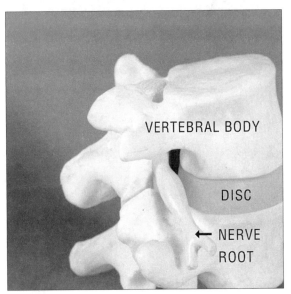

VERTEBRAL BODY

DISC

← NERVE ROOT

Figure 2.5: Two vertebrae

Through this canal runs the bundle of nerves that extends from the head to the pelvis—the spinal cord.

Between each pair of vertebrae are two small openings through which the left and right spinal nerves leave the spinal canal (Fig. 2.5). Among other things, these nerves give power to the muscles and give sensation to the skin. It is through the spinal nerves that you can direct movement and feel temperature, pressure, and pain. These sensations are not just normal parts of life; they also provide a natural alarm system: they warn you that a bodily structure is about to sustain some damage or has already been damaged.

In the lower part of the spine, some of the left and right spinal nerves combine to form the left and right sciatic nerves, which serve the legs. When these nerves are compressed or irritated, they can cause pain in the leg. The pain often extends below the knee. Pain extending from the lower back to below the knee is called sciatica.

Between the spool-like vertebrae are special structures, called discs, made out of cartilage, a dense connective tissue capable of withstanding considerable pressure. In the human body, there are three types of cartilage: *hyaline cartilage*, *elastic cartilage*, and *fibrocartilage*. The type found in the spine is fibrocartilage.

Intervertebral discs are special cartilage structures between the vertebrae. Just as the vertebrae are similar to spools, the discs are similar to rubber washers, round and made of a flexible material; unlike many washers, however, they don't have a hole in the middle.

The semifluid center of the disc is called the *nucleus pulposus*, "nucleus" for short. Surrounding the nucleus is a cartilage ring, called the *annulus* or *annular ligament*.

The discs are the shock absorbers of the spine. They are flexible enough that they can alter their shape, allowing one vertebra to move on another and allowing movement of the back as a whole.

The vertebrae and discs of the lower back form the lumbar spine and are linked by a series of joints. Each joint is held together by soft tissues that surround it. These tissues are reinforced by *ligaments*, tough bands of fibrous connective tissue. The ligaments that reinforce the capsule that surrounds a spinal joint are like guy wires that support an outdoor television antenna by pulling on it and attaching it to the roof. The spinal ligaments strengthen the joint and limit its movement to certain directions.

Then there are the muscles, which lie over one or more joints of the lower back. The muscles extend upward to the trunk and downward to the pelvis. At each end, each muscle becomes a tendon, which attaches the muscle to one or more bones. When a muscle contracts, it causes movement in one or more joints.

BETTER TO BE A QUADRUPED THAN A HUMAN?

Humans descended from four-legged animals but in most ways are more advanced. Few lions or monkeys are good chess players. But, when contrasted to humans, lions and monkeys also have spines that are far less likely to become painful. In animals that walk on all fours, the weight of the body is distributed evenly over the four legs. Most of the time the spine is held in a more or less horizontal position. The forces that compress the human spine simply do not exist.

In human beings, however, the spine is held in a more or less vertical position—at least during waking and working hours. When you are upright, the lumbar spine bears the weight of the entire body above it. This weight compresses the spine. The lumbar spine also transmits this weight to the pelvis when you sit, and to the feet when you stand, walk, or run.

The lumbar spine, providing a flexible connection between the upper and lower halves of the body, protects the spinal cord. It also has a greater function in weight-bearing in humans than it does in quadrupeds. In the evolution of the horizontal spine posture of animals to the vertical spine posture of man, the discs between the vertebrae have adapted to support heavier weights. In addition, the spinal column has developed a series of curves that ingeniously allow for better shock absorption and flexibility.

LOSS OF THE LORDOSIS

Remember the lordosis? That's the natural inward curve, or hollow, in the small of the back (Fig. 2.1). When you stand upright, the lordosis is naturally present. You lose the lordosis when you sit or bend forward. And if you lose the lordosis often or for long periods or both, you can suffer problems of the lower back. In particular, you can suffer problems in the ligaments that act as guy wires supporting and reinforcing the capsule of tissues that surround and hold together the spinal joints. When these ligaments become fatigued or overstretched, pain often results.

MECHANICAL PAIN

Once you have become familiar with this section and the one titled "Mechanical Lower Back Pain," at the beginning of the next chapter, you will be more than halfway toward solving your back and neck pain problems. Research has shown that the better a person understands the problems that cause back or neck pain, the more effectively the person can treat himself or herself. In particular, the person learns why the exercises in this book are effective and how to do these exercises. Further, he or she is more highly motivated to maintain the exercise program.

Mechanical pain occurs when the joint between two bones anywhere in the body has been placed in a position that overstretches the surrounding ligaments and other soft tissues.

To help understand how easily some mechanical pains can be produced, try this experiment:

1. Slowly bend a finger backward (Fig. 2.6). Bend it until you feel a *strain*. If you leave the finger in the strained position, at first you will feel only minor discomfort. But as time passes, substantial *pain* will eventually develop. Sometimes this will take as long as an hour.
2. Repeat the experiment, but with a change. This time, bend the finger past the point of *strain* until you feel *pain*. The sensation of pain is

immediate. In this case, you have over-stretched, and your pain is acting as an alarm system. It is telling you that to continue movement in the current direction will cause damage.

Figure 2.6: Bend the finger until you feel the strain.

The ligaments and surrounding soft tissues that hold the joint together would be torn, resulting in an ache that would continue even when the finger was at rest. This pain would increase with movement and decline at rest, but it would not cease until some healing had occurred. Healing would take several days but would be prolonged if, day after day, you continued to apply the same strains to the finger.

Just as one can experience pain or damage in the finger, one can suffer pain or damage in the back or neck. Holding the neck or back in the wrong position can cause a lot of pain, and holding the back or neck in a position past the point of strain will cause injury.

Most people can sit with poor posture for some period of time without suffering damage or pain. But over time—during a single afternoon or after years of poor posture—the result in most people will eventually be pain and stiffness in the back or neck or both.

We are already doing our best to cause ourselves back and neck trouble. But we are not without help. Our accomplices in the effort to cause ourselves pain through poor posture are the manufacturers of furniture in homes and seats in motor vehicles. Examples of stationary furniture can be found in the home and in the office: kitchen chairs, dining room chairs, lounge chairs, couches, and sofas.

Furniture that moves generally is attached to a car or van or truck. The most common culprit is the car seat. Whether it sits still or moves along at freeway speeds, your seating furniture is probably doing its best to hurt your back and neck.

Bad chairs and bad car seats seem to have been designed by people who own too many rulers: there are too many straight lines. But people's backs and necks contain curves. In particular, there is the lumbar lordosis, which must be maintained if back pain is to be prevented. A seat back that is straight does nothing to maintain the lordosis, and it encourages you to sit in the very slouch that, unfortunately, you are quite capable of producing by yourself.

In addition to having seat backs that are straight, most bad chairs and seats have one other thing in common: they slant backward. Such chairs don't just make it nearly impossible to maintain good posture; these chairs almost *mandate* that the sitter become a sloucher.

But there are alternatives.

First, you can look for good chairs and good car seats. In every case, whether in an office or an automobile, good seats will include an outward curve near the bottom of the seat back. If it is in the right position or if it is adjustable to the right position, this curve will fit into the lordosis, supporting it. Second, if you are stuck with a chair or car seat that looks better than it feels, you can still do something about it. In particular, you can add something to provide the support your lower back needs. For the back, the best device to add is a firm foam rubber lumbar roll.

Certain lumbar rolls are especially effective in helping to avert and treat pain and stiffness in the back. The best design is found not only in the roll's shape but in the precise density and quality of the foam rubber it contains. The best type of lumbar roll comes with an adjustable strap that fits around the back of most any chair or car seat. Until you can get yourself a lumbar roll, try rolling up a bath towel or beach towel or even using a paper towel roll.

Although the lumbar roll of course fits into the lumbar spine, it helps the cervical spine too. It is the opposite of a pain in the neck: it helps to *avoid* a pain in the neck. In supporting the lower back, the lumbar support helps straighten the spine. This in turn naturally causes the posture of the neck to improve, so that the neck is more in a straight line with the rest of the spine. As the neck becomes more in line with the spine, the head retracts. The neck itself is therefore in a more healthful position, and it is not straining by supporting a head that is protruding forward.

There are also well-designed rolls for the neck, called cervical rolls. They are smaller than the lumbar roll but also made of a special foam rubber. The cervical roll is designed to provide proper support of the neck when you lie down to rest or sleep.

Remember, by correcting your lower back posture you also begin the correction of your neck posture. Then, when you simply tuck in your chin while keeping your head and eyes level, your head and neck will be in the proper position, and you will be on your way to stopping your pain.

The better the posture of your back, neck, and head, the faster your pain will go away.

ANATOMY AND EXERCISE

In Chapter 5, you will learn the seven simple exercises that will help you rapidly stop your back symptoms. In Chapter 12, you will learn the seven simple exercises that will help you quickly eliminate your neck pain. In Chapter 21, there are six simple exercises for the shoulder that offer the same benefit. But it may help you to understand the anatomy behind the exercises.

Not all exercises in this book work in the same way, but many are designed to change the shape of the distorted disc. The distortion is often *posterior*, meaning there is a bulge toward the back of the nucleus of the disc and in the back of the annulus, the outer wall that surrounds the nucleus. The bulge causes pain either because the annulus itself contains nerves or because the bulging disc pushes on the spinal nerves. Many of the exercises put the sufferer in "extension," the opposite of "flexion," the forward-bent posture that caused the distortion. Extension causes a tilt in certain adjacent vertebrae, reducing the space between the back parts. This pushes the disc nucleus *anteriorly*, or forward. In this situation, you can move the nucleus easily, like a person with wet hands squeezing a bar of soap. The forward movement of the disc reduces or eliminates the posterior bulge. The result? Your pain is gone.

3 BACK PROBLEMS

MECHANICAL LOWER BACK PAIN

If an engineer were to determine which part of the back was subjected to the greatest mechanical stress, he or she would name the part of the spine just above the pelvis—the lumbar spine. The lower the part of the spine, the more weight it supports. Below the lumbar spine are the *coccyx* and *sacrum*, whose vertebrae don't move and therefore cannot be placed in the wrong position. But the vertebrae of the *lumbar* spine do move and can move into the wrong position; in particular, they can lose their lordosis (their inward curve). In naming the lumbar spine as the focus of the greatest mechanical stress, the engineer would be right, because the lumbar spine is the lowest part of the spine that can move and because statistics show that back problems arise more often in the lower back than in any other part of the spine.

People once believed that pain in the back and neck was caused by drafts, chills, or the weather. But we now know that it is generally caused by mechanical strains of the type described in the previous chapter.

Many people think back and neck pain is caused by muscle strain. Occasionally this is the case. Muscles can indeed be overstretched or injured. But this requires a considerable amount of force and does not happen often. Moreover, muscles usually heal very rapidly and seldom cause pain lasting for more than a week or two.

In fact, most pain in the back and neck is caused by prolonged overstretching of ligaments and other surrounding soft tissues. Just as pain arises in the overstretched finger, pain can arise in the back and neck when ligaments are overstretched.

The most common cause of pain from overstretching is *poor posture.* Whenever you remain in a relaxed position, whether standing, sitting, or lying down, prolonged overstretching can easily occur.

Most people slouch. That's the bad news, but it's also the good news. If the problem was caused only by another person or by a disease, there might be little you could do to prevent it. But since you are the cause, you have control over the problem.

More good news: the strain brought on by prolonged overstretching can easily be avoided. And once you have read this book, you not only will know that you must take responsibility for your posture, but you also will know how to maintain good posture. Further, you will know how to exercise to eliminate pain.

Another source of significant lower back and neck pain is severe overstretching of supporting ligaments. Severe overstretching may occur when an outside force places an excessive strain on the back or neck. This type of strain can occur through a collision in a contact sport, from a fall while playing tennis, or while lifting excessive weight. Other examples of damaging forces are auto accidents and industrial accidents. None of these types of injury can easily be avoided, as they typically occur unexpectedly, without warning signs.

When soft tissues surrounding a joint are overstretched, it is usually the ligaments that first cause pain. Overstretching of the spinal joints causes special problems, because the ligaments that surround these joints also act as retaining walls for the spinal discs. As explained, these discs are the shock absorbers of the spine. Overstretching the spinal ligaments can affect the discs. This may affect the intensity of the pain you feel, the distribution of the pain, and the behavior of the pain. The pain may become better or worse with certain movements or positions.

Sometimes the ligament is injured to such an extent that the disc loses its ability to absorb shock and its outer wall (annulus) is weakened. Once the outer wall is weakened, the soft inside of the disc (the nucleus) bulges outward, often pressing on the spinal nerves and causing pain. Sometimes mere distortion of the outer wall causes pain without impinging on the spinal nerve, because the annulus itself contains nerves.

In extreme cases, the nucleus will burst through this outer wall, which may cause severe pain. If the disc bulges far enough backward, it will press painfully on the sciatic nerve. This can cause pain or other problems (numbness, a sensation of "pins and needles," weakness) to be felt far from the source of trouble—as far away as the lower leg or foot.

If the disc nucleus bulges excessively, the disc may become severely distorted. This will cause the vertebrae to tilt forward or to one side and will prevent the vertebrae from lining up properly during movement. In this case, some movements will be blocked partially or completely, and any movement may cause acute pain.

When acute back pain develops, people often stand with the trunk off center or bent forward. If you experience a sudden onset of pain and, following this, are unable to straighten up or move the back properly, it is likely you have some bulging in the disc nucleus. As bad as this may sound, *this need not be cause for alarm.* The exercises in this book are carefully designed to reduce any disturbance of this nature.

If you have caused damage to soft tissues, you will feel some pain until your healing is complete and your function is fully restored. During the healing process it is important that you avoid movements that pull the healing surfaces apart. For example, if you have overstretched the ligaments of the lower back by bending forward, it is likely that any repetition of this movement will continue to open and separate the healing tissues, and this will delay healing. If, on the other hand, you avoid bending forward and instead retain the hollow (the lumbar lordosis) in the lower back, the damaged surfaces will remain together and healing will not be interrupted. In the same way, if your pain is in the neck, it is important that you avoid bending your neck forward and instead retain the smaller hollow (the cervical lordosis) in your neck.

To illustrate, let's again use the finger, but in a different way. Instead of focusing on overstretching the finger, let's imagine that you have cut your finger across the back of the knuckle. If you were to bend the injured finger joint every day, you would open up the wound and delay healing. But if you were to keep the finger straight for about a week, you would allow the healing surfaces to stay together, and complete healing would result. Once healing was complete, you could bend the finger without risking further damage. Similarly, if you maintain the correct posture and allow your back or neck to heal, you will be able to resume normal bending motion without damage or pain.

But there's more. When tissues heal, they form scar tissue, which is less elastic than normal tissue and tends to shorten over time. If shortening has occurred, movement may stretch the scars and cause pain. Unless appropriate exercises are performed to restore normal flexibility, the healed tissues may become a continuous source of pain or stiffness, or both, in the back or neck. Such problems may persist for years. Even though the original damage has repaired, the scar itself may restrict movement and cause pain when over-stretched.

Where Is the Pain Felt?

The location of pain caused by lower back problems varies from one person to another. In a first attack of back pain, the pain is usually felt at or around the beltline. It may be felt in the center of the back (Fig. 3.1) or just to one side (Fig. 3.2). Usually, the pain declines within a few days.

In later attacks, pain may extend as far as the buttock (Fig. 3.3). In still later episodes, the pain may go all the way to the back or outside of the thigh and on down to the knee (Fig. 3.4). It may even extend to the ankle or foot (Fig. 3.5). Less frequently, pain may be felt in the front of the thigh, down to the knee (Fig. 3.6).

The pain may vary with your movements or with the positions in which you place your body. Its intensity may change. Or its location may vary. For example, one movement may result in buttock pain, while another may eliminate the pain in the buttock, only for the pain to relocate to the lower back.

If your problem is severe, you may have not only pain but other symptoms. In particular, you may experience significant numbness in the lower leg or find that you have muscular weakness in the same place.

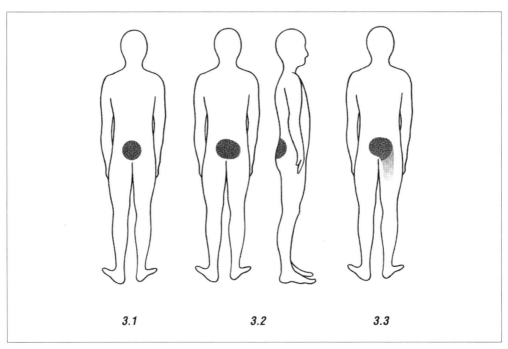

Figures 3.1–3.3: Sites of pain caused by lower back problems

Figures 3.4–3.6: Sites of pain caused by lower back problems

WHO CAN PERFORM SELF-TREATMENT?

Most people with back pain will benefit from the advice in this book. And most people with this pain can immediately start our exercise program—provided that they follow the precautions below. The McKenzie Method program is generally effective, but it is not for every person. It is safe for all, provided that users observe this book's precautions and answer the questions accurately.

Once you start the exercises, carefully observe whether your pain is getting better, getting worse, or staying the same, and whether the location of the pain is changing.

In particular, if your pain was getting worse before you started the exercises and does not improve after the first two days, *seek advice from a health professional* such as a physician, physical therapist, or chiropractor.

In any of the following situations, *do not begin our exercise program* without first consulting a health professional:

- If you have severe pain in the leg below the knee and you experience sensations of weakness, numbness, or "pins and needles" in a foot and the toes.
- If your lower back problems followed a recent severe accident.
- If, following a recent severe episode of back pain, you have developed bladder problems.
- If you are generally feeling unwell in conjunction with the attack of lower back pain (that is, if you have symptoms other than back pain that began around the same time as the back pain).

To help you determine whether you can treat your lower back pain successfully without help from a health professional, please answer the following questions:

YES   NO

- Are there periods in the day—even as short as ten minutes—when you have no pain? ☐ ☐

	YES	NO
• Is the pain confined to areas above the knee?	☐	☐
• Are you generally worse when sitting for prolonged periods or when standing up from the sitting position?	☐	☐
• Are you generally worse during or right after prolonged bending or stooping, as when making a bed, vacuuming, ironing, gardening, or laying concrete?	☐	☐
• Are you generally worse when getting up in the morning, but improve after about a half hour?	☐	☐
• Are you generally worse when inactive and better when on the move?	☐	☐
• Are you generally better when walking?	☐	☐
• Are you generally better when lying facedown? When testing this, you may feel worse for the first few minutes but then feel better; in this case, the answer to this question is yes.	☐	☐
• Have you had several episodes of lower back pain over the past months or years?	☐	☐
• Between episodes, are you able to move fully in all directions without pain?	☐	☐
• Between episodes, are you pain free?	☐	☐
• If you have pain in the buttocks or the upper or lower leg, does it sometimes stop completely, even though you may still have pain in the back?	☐	☐

If you answered yes to all the questions, you are an ideal candidate for the self-treatment program outlined in this book. But we're not hard graders here: there are twelve questions above, and if you answered yes to four or more of them, you have a good chance of benefiting from the program and you should begin it.

Even if you answered yes to fewer than four of the questions, it's possible you will benefit from the program. But to determine whether this is the case, consult a health professional trained in or, ideally, credentialed in the McKenzie Method. This provider can help you determine whether you can start the program or if, instead of our program (or in addition to it), you require a form of specialized treatment that only a health professional can provide. To obtain the names of credentialed members and associates of the McKenzie Institute, please see Appendix A, "How to Find a McKenzie-Trained Health Care Practitioner," which appears at the back of this book.

It is also possible, if you answered yes to fewer than four of the questions, that at least for the moment the distortion in the affected joint is too great to be reduced effectively by self-treatment alone. In that case, ideally you will see a practitioner trained in the McKenzie Method.

4 COMMON CAUSES OF LOWER BACK PAIN

POSTURAL CAUSES

The most common cause of lower back pain is postural stress. For this reason, lower back pain frequently is brought on by sitting for a long time in a poor position (Fig. 4.1), by prolonged bending in a bad working position (Fig. 4.2), by heavy lifting (Fig. 4.3), by relaxing improperly after vigorous activity, or by standing (Fig. 4.4) or lying down for a long time in a poor position. When you look carefully at the accompanying photographs, you will see that the lower back is rounded and that the all-important lordosis—the inward curve or hollow in the lumbar spine—has disappeared.

Unfortunately, many people lose the lordosis much of the time each day and seldom if ever increase it to its very maximum. If you reduce the lordosis for long periods at a time, year in and year out, and you never properly restore it, you will eventually lose your ability to form the hollow. The clinical experience of countless health professionals has demonstrated that a flattened lower back is often associated with chronic lower back problems.

When they walk or run, most people naturally have a lordosis in the lower back. As a result, these activities frequently help to relieve lower back pain.

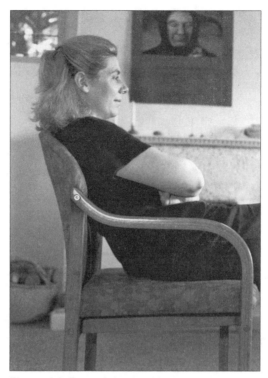

Figure 4.1: Poor sitting position

Figure 4.2: Bad working position

Figure 4.3: Poor lifting technique

Figure 4.4: Standing in poor position

Also, when we are standing, the lordosis naturally is present. But in some individuals, when the standing posture is maintained for a long time, the lordosis becomes excessive and pain will result.

But of all the many postural stresses that can result in pain, by far the worst is poor sitting posture. A poor sitting posture may by itself produce lower back pain. Once lower back problems have developed, a poor sitting posture will in all likelihood perpetuate or worsen these problems.

Other frequent causes of back pain include poor standing postures and poor lying postures. You may know this already, because you may already have found that your back pain appears only if you stand for long periods or only after you get into bed. Pain that behaves in this way frequently is caused by poor posture alone. If this is your situation, you're in luck, because this type of pain can easily be eliminated.

If you have poor posture in sitting, standing, or lying down, you will not have pain as long as you avoid prolonged overstretching. If pain does develop, it's an almost certain indication that you have poor posture and that you must immediately take steps to correct it. Once you have determined what your postural problem is and how to correct it, you should not have to seek assistance from a health professional every time postural pain arises; rather, you should be able to treat yourself rapidly, easily, and effectively.

Consequences of Postural Neglect

Some people who habitually adopt poor posture remain unaware that their posture is causing their back pain. These people experience back pain throughout their lifetime simply because they do not have the information needed to correct the postural faults.

When pain stemming from bad posture is first felt, it is easily eliminated if one merely corrects one's posture. But if time passes and posture is not corrected, the habitual poor posture causes changes in the structure and shape of the joints. As a result, excessive wear occurs in the joints and the joints age prematurely. As a further consequence, the effects of poor posture can be just as severe and just as harmful as the effects of an injury.

Those of us who permit poor posture to persist throughout our lifetimes become bent and stooped as the aging process develops. If we are in this situation, and we are called upon to straighten and stand erect, we cannot do so, much as we might like to. For many of us in this situation, if we are asked to turn the head, we cannot do this either. Our mobility is now so impaired that we appear to others to be old, because we exhibit the posture and mobility problems of the elderly.

Stooped posture and restrictions in mobility are the *visible* effects of poor posture that has become habitual. But there are also secondary consequences to the *organs* that may be even more severe, invisible though they are to others. As the back becomes bent, the lungs may become constricted, which may affect our breathing. The stomach and other internal organs may be deprived of their correct support and may function less effectively than otherwise would be the case.

The typical person believes that the bent, stooped posture seen in so many of our older friends and relatives is an inevitable consequence of aging. This is not the case. And I believe the time to commence preventive action is *now*. If only *once a day* we stand fully erect and bend fully backward, we need never lose the ability to perform those actions and therefore we need never become bent, stooped, and impaired in how we look and in how our bodies function internally.

SITTING FOR LONG PERIODS

Poor posture in sitting is by far the most common cause of pain and stiffness in the back and, for that matter, in the neck. Most everyone spends a great deal of time sitting: even if you do not spend most of your day behind a desk, you probably spend much of your evening in an easy chair or on a couch. *Most* people who sit for long periods will eventually develop poor posture in sitting. This is because when you sit in a particular position for even a few minutes, the muscles that support your lower back and your neck become tired. When they become tired, you relax, placing yourself in a position of poor posture.

Your body sags. You slouch in a chair, adopting a position that is still sitting but is somewhere between sitting straight up and lying down. As a result, you typically lose the lordosis in the back and the lordosis in the neck.

If you stay in a slouched sitting posture long enough, your ligaments will become overstretched and pain and stiffness will result. Worse, once the slouched sitting posture has become a habit and is maintained most of the time, it may also cause distortion of the nucleus of the discs in the vertebral joints. (A distorted disc is one that has lost its normal shape; typically, it bulges in one direction or another.) Once this occurs, pain will come not only from certain positions but from certain movements.

Poor sitting posture may itself produce lower back pain. And, regardless of the original cause, once lower back pain or stiffness has developed, poor sitting posture will perpetuate or worsen the problem.

It follows that people with office jobs that involve a lot of sitting easily develop lower back problems, because many sit with a rounded back—a back not maintaining the lordosis—for hours on end. If you are an office worker, you may go through the following stages of gradually increasing back problems, unless you take steps to rectify the cause.

- At first, you may experience lower back discomfort only while sitting for a prolonged period, or on standing up after sitting down. In this case, the pain is caused by the overstretching of soft tissues, and it takes only a few seconds for the tissues to recover. At this stage, the pain exists only for a short time.
- At a later stage, you will find that on standing up you have increased pain, and you must walk carefully for a short distance before you can straighten up fully. Now it is likely that some distortion has occurred in one of the lumbar discs: prolonged sitting has led to minor distortion of a disc, and the disc needs a few minutes to recover.
- Eventually, you may reach the stage where you frequently experience sharp or agonizing pain on standing and you are unable to straighten up even after walking carefully. If this is the case, there is a major distortion of the affected disc, which cannot regain its normal shape quickly enough to allow pain-free movement. Instead, whenever a movement is attempted, the disc bulge increases the strain on the surrounding tissues, which are already overstretched. In addition, the disc bulge may pinch the sciatic nerve, which may cause pain and other symptoms in the leg.

Figure 4.5a–b: Poorly designed seating

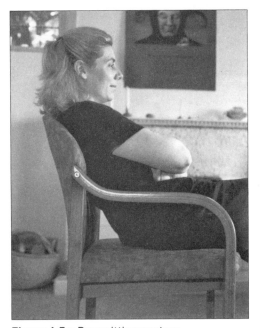

Figure 4.5c: Poor sitting posture

Environmental Factors

We can blame ourselves for a lot, but if you would prefer to also blame others, this is your opportunity. Designers are out to get you! The design of seating—whether found in transportation, business settings, or the home—is focused more on sales than on posture. More specifically, the common designs seem focused on appearance and an immediate sense of physical comfort, even if in the long run pain and stiffness and even injury are the result.

Seating design contributes to our poor postural habits. Chairs rarely give adequate support to the lower back. Unless you make a conscious effort to sit correctly, you are more or less forced to sit badly (Figs. 4.5a–c).

Ideally, the backs of all chairs would provide a lumbar support so that the lordosis, which is naturally present in standing, is also maintained while sitting (Figs. 4.6a and 4.6b). But rarely do seat designers include this support.

Equally important, furniture in offices and factories should be adapted to individual requirements. For example, if you are a desk worker, you must make sure that the seat of your chair has the correct height. This means that as you sit, your feet should rest flat on the floor and your thighs should remain horizontal without your having to press on the seat.

Figure 4.6a: Well-designed typist or secretarial chair

Figure 4.6b: Well-designed lounge chair

The desk itself must also be the correct height. If the surface you lean on is too low, you will slouch forward and lose the lordosis. If the desk surface is too low, raise the desk by using wooden blocks.

Finally, armrests must be positioned in such a way that, when you use them, your shoulders are neither raised nor lowered too much. Your shoulders are at the wrong height if you feel discomfort in them after ten to twenty minutes.

Armrests also should allow your chair to be pulled under your desk so that you can sit with your stomach held gently against the front of the desk. This will prevent you from leaning over and losing the lordosis while you perform desk tasks.

Until furniture designers understand and defer to the requirements of the human frame, we will continue to suffer from their neglect.

Although the poor design of furniture contributes to the development of lower back problems, equal blame must be placed upon the individual who uses a chair improperly. If we do not know how to sit correctly, even the best chairs will not prevent us from slouching. On the other hand, once we have learned the correct concepts, poorly designed chairs will not have such a detrimental effect on our sitting posture.

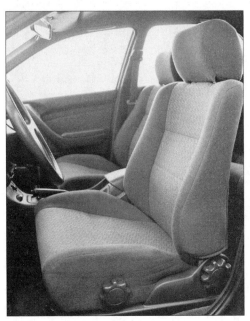

Figure 4.7: The McKenzie seat

Years ago, the Toyota Motor Corporation in New Zealand asked the McKenzie Institute International to provide expertise to assist the company in the design of new seats for a variety of its vehicles sold in that country. From this cooperative venture emerged a seat with outstanding qualities. It combined spinal support and driver stability (Fig. 4.7). The seat met with universal consumer approval, especially when used for extended trips. Eventually Toyota in New Zealand changed the design of its cars and moved to a different seat design.

Similarly, the McKenzie Institute has become involved in the design of furniture for relaxing in the home. It is a goal of the institute that well-designed home furniture be widely available and affordable.

Sitting Correctly for Long Periods

If you have pain resulting from factors other than just poor posture, you may need to do more than correct your posture. You may need to perform special exercises. In this chapter, I am describing only the exercises required to reduce postural stress and to obtain postural correction. In later chapters, you will find exercises for relief of pain and increase of function in both the back and the neck.

In order to avoid the development of lower back pain due to prolonged poor sitting, it is necessary that you (1) sit correctly and (2) interrupt prolonged sitting at regular intervals.

Correcting the Sitting Posture

From now on, you must pay a lot of attention to your sitting posture. I know this will strike some of you as bad news, or even unnecessary news. The fact is, however, that you can get used to paying more attention to your sitting posture—used to it in such a way that it does not interfere with your life.

Further, the fact is that if you don't take the fairly minimal trouble to correct your sitting posture, you may pay a price far more costly than a relatively simple change in behavior: you may develop back pain that is severe or even disabling, and you may develop the irreversible bent-over posture associated with the elderly.

You may have had the habit of sitting slouched for many years without lower back pain, but once you have developed lower back pain problems, you must no longer sit in the old way. The slouched posture will only perpetuate the overstretching and distortion of the joints.

In order to sit correctly, you must first learn *how to form a lordosis* in the lower back while sitting. Therefore, you must become fully practiced in what I call the "slouch-overcorrect" procedure. Once you have achieved this, you must learn *how to maintain a lordosis* in the lower back while sitting for long periods.

Figure 4.8: Extreme of slouched sitting position

How to Form a Lordosis while Seated: The Slouch-Overcorrect Procedure

You must sit on a stool of chair height. If a stool is unavailable, the edge of a chair will do. Once seated, allow yourself to slouch completely (Fig. 4.8). Now you are ready to commence the slouch-overcorrect procedure.

Relax for a few seconds in the slouched position. Then draw yourself up and accentuate the lordosis as far as possible (Fig. 4.9). This is the extreme of the good sitting position. Hold yourself in this position for a few seconds.

Now return to the fully relaxed position (Fig. 4.8).

Do these movements as you *slowly* think or say the words "pressure on, pressure off." Remain in the

Figure 4.9: Accentuating the lordosis

first position during "pressure on," the second position during "pressure off." Combining the words with the movements helps you to hold each position for the right amount of time and to establish a rhythm. The technique of slowly thinking or speaking the words "pressure on, pressure off" can be used with all the McKenzie exercises for the back, neck, and shoulder that involve multiple movements.

In the exercise to form a lordosis, the movement from the slouched position to the upright position should be done in such a way that you move rhythmically from the extreme of the bad to the extreme of the good sitting posture.

CASE HISTORY: NURSING HERSELF BACK TO HEALTH

Greta, a forty-one-year-old nurse, works on a surgical floor at a hospital in Indiana. Her doctor diagnosed her with lumbar radiculitis, meaning she had inflammation of a lumbar nerve root. She had lower back pain as well as leg pain going all the way to her heel. Greta had had these symptoms for six months and they were getting worse. She had suffered no injury and had no idea why she had back pain.

The symptoms had begun in her left buttock. Her lower back pain was constant and her leg symptoms intermittent. She had limited range of motion in the back. She was unable to sit for long periods and unable to sleep through the night.

Using McKenzie postural techniques, including the use of a lumbar roll and the slouch-overcorrect exercise, Greta was able to sit more comfortably and for longer periods. She also benefited from Back Exercise 3, Extension in Lying. This greatly reduced her leg symptoms.

A week after starting with the McKenzie Method, Greta's symptoms had centralized, so that they were only in the left buttock. That is, her leg pain was completely gone. She was able to sleep through the night. She had improved range of motion in the lumbar spine.

About ten days later, she progressed to Back Exercise 5, Flexion in Lying, but kept up with Back Exercise 3 as well. A week later, Greta had no symptoms and full range of motion. She progressed to Back Exercise 7, Flexion in Standing, instead of in lying down, and kept up with Exercise 3. She remained pain free.

Perform the exercise ten or fifteen times per session. Repeat the sessions three times per day, preferably once in the morning, once around noon, and once in the evening. In addition, do the exercise whenever pain arises as a result of sitting poorly. Each time you repeat the cycle of movements (slouch-upright-slouch), be sure the movements are performed to the maximum possible degree, particularly in the upright position.

Maintaining the Lordosis

You have just learned how to find the *extreme of the good sitting posture.* It is not possible to sit in this way for long periods, because it causes considerable strain and, if maintained for excessive periods, might actually cause pain. To sit comfortably and correctly, you must sit in a way that is not as upright as the position of extreme good posture. To find the correct position, you must first sit with your lower back in extreme lordosis (Fig. 4.9) and then release the last 10 percent of the lordosis strain. At the same time, take care to ensure that you do not allow the lower back to flatten (Fig. 4.10).

Now you have reached the correct sitting posture, which can be maintained for any length of time. When sitting like this, you maintain the lordosis of the lower back with your own muscular effort. It requires constant attention and constant effort, and you cannot fully relax. And whenever you sit on a seat without a back, you must sit in this way.

The Lumbar Roll

Relatively few chairs' seat backs provide adequate support for the lower back. For this reason, for people with ongoing back problems, a portable lumbar roll is essential equipment. When sitting on a seat that has a back, you will find that a lumbar roll will facilitate the maintenance of a correct lordosis and correct posture.

Figure 4.10: Extreme of good sitting position: less lordosis strain creates correct sitting posture.

Figure 4.11: Lumbar roll

A lumbar roll (Fig. 4.11) is a fat, cylindrical-shaped support made mostly of foam rubber that is designed specifically for the lower back. Without this support, the lower back will slouch whenever you are distracted or stop concentrating on anything other than holding the lordosis actively with your own muscles. For instance, if you must focus on talking, reading, writing, watching TV, or driving your car, chances are you will lose the lordosis and slouch into bad posture—unless you use a lumbar roll. You may be concentrating on being a brilliant conversationalist, but your lumbar roll is a faithful little fellow, and he's focused on one thing: maintaining your lordosis.

To avoid the slouching that ordinarily would occur as you concentrate on something other than your lordosis and your posture, you must place a lumbar roll in the small of your back at the level of your beltline whenever you sit in a standard chair (Fig. 4.12), a car (Fig. 4.13), or an office chair (Figs. 4.14a and 4.14b).

Figure 4.12: Use of lumbar roll to correct poor chair design

You may purchase a lumbar roll specifically

made for the above purpose from the authorized firm listed in Appendix B of this book. You will need to provide your waist measurement and your weight.

The lumbar roll should be no more than four to five inches (about ten to thirteen centimeters) in diameter before being compressed. It should be filled with foam rubber of moderate density so that when compressed its diameter reduces to about one and a half inches (about four centimeters).

A regular seat-back cushion does not serve the same purpose as a lumbar roll because it is the wrong shape and does not provide adequate pressure at the key level of the lower back. Do not rely on a regular cushion for long-term use, but it may be of some assistance in an emergency. Also inappropriate for the long term but of possible value in a pinch is a rolled-up bath towel or beach towel or even a roll of paper towels.

Figure 4.13: Use of lumbar roll to correct poor car seat design

The first aim of this part of the program is to restore the correct posture. The second goal is to maintain it. It may take up to a week to master this fully. *As a rule, pain that is due to bad posture will decrease as your sitting posture improves*, and once you maintain the correct posture, you will have no pain at all. In the first few weeks, if you allow yourself to slouch while sitting, the pain will readily come back. Eventually, though, you will remain completely pain free even when you forget your posture. Even so, you should never again allow yourself to sit in a slouched position for long periods.

The first few times you use these procedures to correct your sitting posture, you will experience some new pains. These will be different from your original pain, and you may feel them in new places. New pains result from performing new exercises and maintaining new positions. They should be expected, and they will wear off in a few days—*if* you continue to correct your posture on a regular basis. Once you have become used to sitting correctly, you will *enjoy* it. And soon you will notice the reduction or absence of pain and you will simply sit with more comfort. On the other hand, if you slouch, pain can return.

Figure 4.14a: Poor office chair design uncorrected

Figure 4.14b: Poor office chair design corrected by lumbar roll

At first, many patients who have become used to sitting correctly do not even notice their symptoms have gone away. Only later does the person realize that his or her back has become so pain free that he or she is no longer thinking about it. Once you are used to sitting with the correct posture, you will automatically choose chairs that allow you to sit correctly.

> **RULE:** When sitting for long periods, you must sit correctly: with the lower back in a moderate lordosis. Whenever your seat has a back, you must use a lumbar roll to support your lower back.

In 1988, the McKenzie Institute commissioned a study to examine the effects of sitting with and without a lumbar roll. One group used the roll; one group didn't. Those using the roll were required to use it at home, at the office, and when driving. The results showed conclusively that the patients using a lumbar roll whenever sitting experienced much less pain than those not using the roll.

Regularly Interrupting Prolonged Sitting

Traveling for long distances by car, bus, or plane may cause a gradual and progressive attack of lower back pain or aggravate existing problems. This is the case especially when you sit in a cramped seat and do not take regular breaks that would permit you to restore your lordosis. After an uninterrupted car ride of even a few hours, nearly everyone will notice some stiffness or discomfort in the lower back. If you already have back problems, such a journey may be a risky experience for you. If you are the driver, the risk is even greater than if you are a passenger.

In order to minimize the risks of prolonged sitting, you must interrupt sitting at regular intervals and *before pain starts*. For example, during long car trips, once an hour you should stop the car, get out, bend backward five or six times (see Back Exercise 4 in the next chapter), and then walk around for a few minutes. This will reduce the pressure within the discs and relieve the stresses on the surrounding tissues.

As long as airlines continue to provide seating seemingly calculated to damage the human spine, you should take action when traveling on planes as well. When flying long distances, regularly stand up and walk up and down an aisle of the plane. Not only is this important for your back, but it also stimulates circulation in the legs.

Taking breaks during travel, whether in a car or on a plane, will significantly reduce the risk of another episode of back pain.

RULE: When you sit for prolonged periods, regular interruption of the sitting posture is essential to prevent the onset of pain. You can interrupt this posture by standing upright, bending backward five or six times, and walking about for a few minutes. (See Back Exercise 4.)

CASE HISTORY: FURNITURE FACTORY

Isaac, forty-eight, owns a furniture factory in Pennsylvania and is himself one of the furniture makers. He had episodic pain in the right lower back. This resulted from an injury at work suffered while bending over and rotating to the left. He subsequently felt pain when bending, lifting, and sitting.

He had seen a chiropractor, but with little effect. He had been taking the prescription drug Percoset and the over-the-counter medication Aleve.

With the McKenzie Method, he learned to sit correctly at work and while driving and also improved his posture when standing. He also used Back Exercise 3, Extension in Lying, and Back Exercise 4, Extension in Standing. Within two days, his pain was gone. He remained symptom free.

WORKING IN STOOPED POSITIONS

Stooped positions often result in back pain. When you stand with your back straight, the stresses on the discs and ligaments of your lower back are considerably lower than when you stand with your back bent forward. Many activities around the home ordinarily involve bending, for example, gardening, vacuuming, and making a bed (Fig. 4.15). Occupations requiring a prolonged stooped posture are abundant: assembly-line worker, farmworker, bricklayer, electrician, plumber, carpenter, surgeon, nurse. The list goes on and on. People in all these occupations are in most cases required to bend forward for prolonged periods every day (Fig. 4.16). While working with a stooped posture, you are most likely to experience back problems in the first four or five hours of the day.

Figure 4.15: Vacuuming usually involves bending.

In order to minimize the risks involved in prolonged forward bending, interrupt the stooped position at regular intervals. And it is important that you interrupt it *before pain starts*. Stand upright and bend backward five or six times (see Back Exercise 4). This is especially important if you already have developed lower back problems by working in a stooped position. Regular interruption of the stooped position will correct any distortion that may have occurred in the discs and will relieve the stresses on the surrounding tissues.

When this interruption occurs before pain starts, it usually prevents the development of significant lower back pain. *Remember: you are especially at risk in the first half of your day*, so make sure you pay attention to your posture during this period.

Figure 4.16: Prolonged stooped position

RULE: When working in a stooped position, you must regularly interrupt the bent posture in order to prevent the onset of pain. You can do this by standing upright and bending backward five or six times. (See Back Exercise 4.)

LIFTING

Lifting an object with your back rounded (Fig. 4.17a) raises the pressure in your discs to a much higher level than if you were to lift the same object with your body upright and your lordosis present. Research has borne this out. Just as back problems associated with stooped positions seem to occur very frequently in the first four or five hours of the day (because the discs take up fluid while we rest at night), the same is true with lifting. This is the case especially if you lift repeatedly and frequently. If you use an incorrect technique while

Figure 4.17a: Poor lifting technique

lifting a heavy object, you may cause damage and pain, and the pain may be not only sudden but severe.

In order to minimize the risks involved in lifting, always use the correct lifting technique (Figs. 4.17b–f). *Immediately before and after lifting*, stand upright and bend backward five or six times. (See Back Exercise 4.) You should do this especially when a single heavy lift is involved. If you must lift many objects, one after another, frequently interrupt the lifting and repeat the backward-bending exercise. By standing upright and bending backward before lifting, you ensure that, as you begin the lift, there is no distortion already present in the joints of the lower back. This is particularly important if, immediately before you start lifting, you have been in a stooped position or have been sitting for a long period.

For example, many truck drivers drive for

Figure 4.17b–d: Correct lifting technique

hours and hours and then are called upon to remove heavy objects from the back of their truck. A more common example comes when you take a car trip, sit in the car for several hours before stopping, arrive at your destination, and remove heavy objects from the trunk. Whether you're a truck driver or a car passenger, when you've been on the road for a long time, take a moment before lifting. Stand upright and bend backward a few times before and after lifting. By doing so, you will correct any distortion that may have developed in the joints as a result of sitting.

If you are suffering from lower back pain right now, and especially if your pain has been caused by lifting, it is best to completely avoid lifting for a few weeks. This will permit damaged tissues to heal. If it is not possible to avoid lifting, you must at all times use the correct lifting technique and avoid lifting objects that are awkward to handle or heavier than thirty pounds (about fifteen kilograms).

Once you have developed recurrent lower back problems, you should never again handle awkward or heavy objects by yourself. This is true even if you are completely free of pain. In addition, you should become familiar with the correct lifting technique. After some practice with this technique, lifting correctly will become a habit.

Figure 4.17e–f: Correct lifting technique

Correct Lifting Technique

Throughout a lift, you must attempt to retain the lordosis in your lower back (Figs. 4.17b–f). You make the lift by straightening your legs. Avoid using the back as a crane (Fig. 4.17a).

Correct lifting technique involves the following:

- Stand close to the load. Have a firm footing and a wide stance.
- Exaggerate the lordosis.
- As you descend to approach the load, bend your knees and keep your back straight.
- Get a secure grip and hold the load as close to your body as possible.

CASE HISTORY: GETTING A LIFT

Florence is a fifty-eight-year-old cleaning lady who works at a physician's office and who also baby-sits her grandchildren. She lives in Florida. She had distressing lower back pain for two and a half weeks, and had experienced lower back pain off and on for five years. The new episode began when she bent over in her cleaning work. Her pain got worse when she bent, lifted, sat, lay on either side, or walked almost any distance. She was also worse in the morning. Her sitting posture was only fair, and she had pain after sitting for long periods.

Back Exercise 3, Extension in Lying, reduced her pain, but only during the exercise. She began doing this exercise five times a day and began using a lumbar roll when sitting. Six days later, her back pain had decreased, and she could walk greater distances before the onset of pain.

She learned to improve her posture through the slouch-overcorrect procedure, and she added this to her exercise program, doing it two to three times a day.

Still, bending and lifting at work continued to bother her. She learned to lift properly, not by bending over but rather by maintaining the lordosis in her lumbar spine and using her quadriceps (upper leg) muscles to lift.

She began to do Back Exercise 4, Extension in Standing, throughout her workday, especially after bending. With the use of the lumbar roll, she found she could sit without pain for longer periods than before.

> She began Back Exercise 5, Flexion in Lying. It caused her no symptoms and no reduction in her ability to extend her spine. She did this exercise two to three times a day, followed by Back Exercise 3, Extension in Lying. Two weeks after beginning to use these two exercises, she was pain free and able to resume all her previous activities.

- Lean back to stay in balance, and lift the load by straightening the knees.
- Make the lift with a steady motion. Don't jerk.
- Once you have become upright and you need to turn the weight, turn it by shifting your feet, not by twisting your lower back.

> **RULE:** When lifting, use the correct lifting technique. In addition, immediately before and after each heavy single lift, stand upright and bend backward five or six times. (See Back Exercise 4.) When you lift repeatedly, perform the same exercise at regular intervals.

RELAXING AFTER VIGOROUS ACTIVITY

Over the years I have heard many people complain that they develop back pain after engaging in activities such as gardening, laying concrete, or even running. It is easy, even logical, to attribute the pain to the activity. After all, one has followed the other. In many cases, one has followed the other repeatedly: every time the person gardens, he or she has a sore lower back afterward. In fact, however, very often it is not the strenuous physical activity that is the culprit.

Very often, following such an activity, we sit and relax. We may collapse into a slouched position in a chair. We may sit on the grass, bent over at the waist. We may stand, out of breath, bent forward at the waist, supporting our upper body by placing our hands on our knees. After a while we feel pain, and we automatically blame the activity that we have just completed.

Instead, we should consider the likelihood that the pain has begun as a result of the posture we adopted *subsequent to the exercise.* If the activity itself had been responsible for the pain, we would have felt some discomfort or pain during the activity. This would have been due to overstretching or injury occurring during the activity. If we had hurt ourselves during exercise, pain would not likely have arisen significantly after the activity (often, pain following exercise takes an hour or so to arise). Rather, it would have occurred immediately, during the activity.

After activity, the joints of the spine undergo a loosening process. If, after exercise, we place the back in an unsupported position for a long period, distortion within the joint readily occurs. This is true whether we sit in a slouched position or we stand, bent forward with our hands on our knees. *Thoroughly exercised joints of the spine distort easily if the spine is placed in a slouched position for a long period.* For more on how pain following an activity often is not caused by the activity itself, see the discussion of sports-related injuries in Chapter 8.

> **RULE:** After vigorous activity, restore and exaggerate the lordosis by standing upright and bending backward five or six times. (See Back Exercise 4.) When you sit down to rest, maintain the lordosis and use a lumbar roll in order to avoid slouching.

PROLONGED STANDING

Some people get lower back pain every time they stand in one place for a long time. The same thing happens when we sit for long periods. In either situation, the muscles that support us tire and relax, allowing us to slouch. When we stand in a relaxed manner, however, the lordosis *becomes excessive* and the lower back hangs in an extreme position.

This position is exactly opposite to that adopted by the spine when we sit in a slouch. It is not possible to stand in this relaxed way for long periods, because the excessive lordosis is a position of strain. If your lower back pain occurs during long periods of standing, you will find relief by correcting your standing posture.

Correcting the Standing Posture

To stand correctly, you must hold your lower back in a position of reduced lordosis. To find this position, first you must stand relaxed. Allow the chest to sag and the abdomen to protrude slightly. This will place the lower lumbar joints in an extreme lordosis.

Next, reduce lordosis by standing as tall as you can. Lift the chest up, pull in your stomach, and tighten your buttocks (Fig. 4.18).

You have now reached the correct standing posture. When standing like this, you reduce the lordosis through your own muscular effort.

To begin with, you will find it difficult to hold this position, but with practice you can learn to stand in the new position for long periods without discomfort.

Figure 4.18: Correct standing posture

LYING DOWN AND RESTING

Some people have lower back pain when they lie resting in certain positions. A relative few have lower back pain only when they lie down. Many people with lower back pain feel worse when they are lying down, and they dread the thought of another night with more back pain and less sleep.

If you have lower back pain only when you are lying down, or if you regularly awake in the morning with a stiff and painful lower back that was not painful the night before, one of two things is probably wrong. Either there is something wrong with the surface on which you are lying or there is something wrong with the position in which you sleep (Figs. 4.19a and 4.19b).

It is a comparatively easy task to correct the surface on which you are

Figure 4.19a–b: Poor lying position

lying, but it is rather difficult to influence the position you adopt while sleeping. Once you are asleep, you may frequently change your position or "toss and turn." Unless a certain position causes so much discomfort that it wakes you up, you will have no idea of the various positions you assume while sleeping.

Many people with back problems are told never to lie facedown while in bed. This can indeed make it difficult to recover from an injury to the *neck*, but there is no evidence whatsoever to suggest that this is harmful to the back. On the contrary, it may well be that your back will stop being painful if you sleep in the facedown position.

If you have not already discovered the effects of lying facedown, you should experiment. Next time you have back pain while lying down, see what effect lying facedown has on your problem. The results will vary from person to person. Certainly there are some lower back problems that are aggravated by lying facedown. And if you have sciatica, lying facedown is nearly always impossible. But for many back sufferers, lying facedown will bring relief.

CASE HISTORY: NUMBNESS AND TINGLING

Rose, seventy-six, from Florida, is a retiree whose physician diagnosed her with lumbar radiculitis (inflammation of a lumbar nerve root). For two months, she'd had lower back pain as well as numbness and tingling in the right leg and foot. Her symptoms came and went but were most often provoked by sitting. Her pain interrupted her sleep.

Back Exercise 3, Extension in Lying, reduced Rose's symptoms in the right leg and foot.

Five days later she had less numbness and tingling in the foot but more of each in the thigh. Using a lumbar roll while sitting had reduced the symptoms in the foot. Per the McKenzie Method, she was sleeping on her stomach, and this further reduced the foot problems.

Two days later Rose was able to sit for longer periods and was sleeping much better, and her leg symptoms had declined dramatically. Back Exercise 3 remained the key one for her.

Four days later, she was sleeping through the night and her foot symptoms were better still. She used the slouch-overcorrect procedure without difficulty and it helped to improve her posture.

Two days later Rose could easily tolerate Back Exercise 5, Flexion in Lying. Five days after that, she was symptom free. She progressed to Back Exercise 7, Flexion in Standing.

She remained free of pain and had full range of motion.

Correcting the Surface for Lying Down

There are two simple ways in which you may be able to reduce strain on your lower back caused by lying on a faulty surface.

The first and most important way is to lie with a supportive lumbar roll around your waist. The roll will support your lower back as you rest, and it will prevent the strain that can develop when you lie on your side or back.

You may purchase a lumbar night roll specifically made for this purpose from the firm mentioned in Appendix B of this book. You will need to supply your waist measurement and your weight.

A good temporary alternative is to use a rolled beach towel or bath towel. Fold the towel in half from end to end, then roll it from the side.

Your goal is to create a roll of about three inches (seven to eight centimeters) in diameter and three feet (about ninety centimeters) in length. Wind the roll around your waist at the level where you normally wear a belt and hold it together in front with a safety pin to ensure that it remains in place. If the towel is not held together properly, the roll may move up or down during your sleep. If the towel has moved to the wrong place, it may actually *increase* your pain during or after sleep.

The diameter and length given above are merely guides: lumbar supports need to fulfill individual requirements, and each person must experiment for himself or herself. You can follow the general rule that when you lie on your side, the roll should fill the natural hollow in the body's shape between the pelvis and the rib cage. The other general rule is that when you lie on your back, the roll should support the lower back, placing it in a moderate lordosis (Figs. 4.20a and 4.20b).

The second way to reduce strain on your lower back is to ensure that your mattress does not sag. The mattress itself should not be too hard. In fact, a soft mattress can be extremely comfortable, provided it is placed on a firm support.

To ensure that your mattress is supported on a firm, hard surface, it is best to experiment by placing it on the floor. Spend three to four nights sleeping with the mattress supported in this manner; this will allow you to determine if poor support for your mattress is the source of your back pain.

Avoid a bed with a wire base. (Commonly used in the 1950s and '60s, this is a base or frame with wires stretched across it and adjusted with bolts.) Use a firm base; a box spring may be used if it is firm and does not sag. Another example of a firm base would be the solid wood base found in a bed frame made to support a mattress alone, as opposed to a metal frame designed to support a box spring and mattress. If a solid base is not readily available, the

Figure 4.20a–b: Lying position corrected by lumbar night roll

effects of a soft box spring can be reduced by inserting slats or a bed board—a rigid piece of plywood—between the box spring and mattress.

The mattress itself may be either of the most common types: innerspring or foam rubber.

If you have tried these suggestions without benefit, consult a health care provider trained in the treatment of lower back pain. Members and associates of the McKenzie Institute are well versed in the management of problems related to lying and resting. It may be that you need special advice regarding the surface on which you lie or the posture you assume while you sleep. It may also be that you need special treatment for your lower back problems.

COUGHING AND SNEEZING

Coughing and sneezing while you are bent forward or sitting may cause a sudden attack of lower back pain or aggravate existing back pain. If you sense the need to cough or sneeze, try to stand upright and bend backward before coughing or sneezing, so that your lower back is hollow—in lordosis—at the moment the cough or sneeze comes. Should you not be able to stand up, at least lean backward, making the best possible lordosis.

5 THE MCKENZIE METHOD EXERCISES FOR THE BACK

GENERAL GUIDELINES AND PRECAUTIONS

The McKenzie back exercise program consists of seven exercises. The McKenzie *neck* exercise program consists of seven different exercises; you will find them in Chapter 12. You'll find the six shoulder exercises in Chapter 21.

Even though there are seven exercises, it is unlikely that in any one session you will need to do more than two. So the exercise program is neither hard nor time-consuming.

The first four back exercises are extension exercises, and the last three are flexion exercises. In regard to the back, *extension* means bending backward, and *flexion* means bending forward.

The purpose of the back exercises is to eliminate pain and, where possible, restore normal function—that is, to regain full mobility in the lower back or as much movement as possible under the circumstances. When you are exercising for pain relief, you move to the edge of the pain or just into the pain, then release the pressure and return to the starting position. But when you are exercising in order to regain lost movement or to reduce stiffness, try to attain the maximum amount of movement; to do this, you may have to move well into the pain.

Postural correction and maintenance of the correct posture should always follow the exercises. Even when you no longer have lower back pain, good postural habits are essential to prevent the recurrence of your problems. These habits, therefore, should be followed for the rest of your life.

THE EXERCISES ARE ONLY PART OF THE MCKENZIE METHOD

Soon we will get to specific exercises that can give you relief promptly or even immediately. But first, let's discuss the benefits of the exercises in general.

Obviously, the McKenzie exercises eliminate or dramatically reduce pain and stiffness. But the McKenzie Method is much more than exercises. And the exercises are much more than extension: some of them involve the opposite movement, flexion.

The McKenzie Method involves instructing back and neck sufferers in how their spine works and how—especially through bad posture in sitting and standing—they are hurting themselves. Consistent with this, it also involves helping people with back or neck pain to correct their daily habits so that they can become pain free.

A further hallmark of the McKenzie Method is that the exercises typically cause more than relief of pain and stiffness; they also cause a *centralization* of pain or stiffness. When symptoms centralize, they move to the center of the spine, or close to the center, where they are almost always more tolerable than at their more distant locations, even though the pain may increase. Back pain that has radiated down the legs, sometimes as far as the feet, becomes localized in or near the center of the lower back; back pain that is felt mostly on the right or left of the lower back becomes localized closer to its center. This is proof that the exercises are effective for the particular back sufferer, and readers doing the exercises should watch for this encouraging effect.

Health professionals worldwide have confirmed my discovery that centralization is the primary indicator of good progress, shows that the exercises will help, and demonstrates that an expert need not be consulted. In most cases, you can make the same determination yourself: if, after doing the exercises for a while, your pain centralizes, you very likely can treat yourself successfully, without relying on health care providers.

Research has shown that in many instances, centralization is as effective as an MRI (magnetic resonance imaging) in determining the nature of a patient's problems. In addition, very recent studies show the McKenzie Method's assessment techniques identify intact discs and demonstrate good progress.

CASE HISTORY: CENTRALIZATION IN TEXAS

Walt is from Texas. He is fifty-four years old and works as an insurance broker. For two months he had intermittent pain in the central and lower left back. This had come on for no apparent reason. It spread to his left buttock and thigh, and the symptoms were worse when he bent forward, sat, rose to stand, coughed, or sneezed. He felt better when he moved, especially when he walked, and especially later in the day.

He had poor sitting posture and a slight loss of range of motion in lumbar extension. His first McKenzie exercise was Back Exercise 3, Extension in Lying. He moved on to Back Exercise 7, Flexion in Standing, which reduced his pain during the exercise but not after. He also learned the McKenzie techniques of postural correction, especially the slouch-overcorrect movements.

Within two days, Walt's back pain had centralized but was more intense. Overall, however, this was a good sign, a sign that he could treat himself successfully with the McKenzie exercises. He continued with Back Exercise 3, about every two hours during the day. Within two more days, his back pain was gone and his range of motion was complete. With continuation of Exercise 3 and other McKenzie extension exercises for the back, he remained free of symptoms.

PAIN INTENSITY AND PAIN MOVEMENT

Read This Section Carefully.

The exercises in this book are not designed to strengthen the muscles of your back. We have found that if we can rid you of pain and return you to normal activity, then in the normal course of events your strength will return.

The exercises are designed to correct any distortion or bulging that may have developed in the joints of the lower back. By reducing the distortion or bulging of the intervertebral disc, we can in turn reduce the level of pain that you experience.

The exercises also will identify for you any movements or postures that are likely to increase the distortion in the joints and therefore delay recovery. In turn, your experience with the exercises will enable you to avoid damaging postures and activities in the future.

You can look for three main effects when performing the exercises:

- First, the exercises may cause the symptoms to disappear. This may occur almost immediately or over the course of one to four weeks.
- Second, they may cause an increase or decrease in the intensity of the pain that you experience.
- Third, they may cause the pain to move from where you usually feel it to some other location. In certain cases, the symptoms first will change location, then decrease in intensity, and finally cease altogether.

Specifically, pain can improve in many ways:

- It can become less intense.
- It can become less frequent.
- You can sustain activity longer before the pain occurs.
- You can move farther before pain begins.
- Constant pain can be replaced by intermittent pain.
- Pain can centralize. (This not only provides for a more comfortable type of pain but predicts a good outcome through the McKenzie exercises.)

Each one of these improvements is an indication that your condition is improving.

The effects of exercise on the intensity or location of pain can sometimes be very rapid. It is possible to reduce the intensity or change the location of back pain after completing as few as ten or twelve movements (that is, as few as two repetitions of a session in which an exercise is done five or six times). Sometimes, the pain will completely disappear with just that small amount of effort.

In order to determine whether the exercise program is working effectively for you, it is very important that you observe closely any changes in the intensity or location of your pain. You may notice that as a result of the exercises, the pain, originally felt across the lower back, to one side of the spine, or in one buttock or thigh, moves toward the center of the lower back. In other words, you may notice that your pain *localizes or centralizes.*

Centralization of pain (Fig. 5.1) that occurs as you exercise is a good sign. If your pain moves to the midline of the spine and away from areas where it is usually felt, this means you are exercising correctly and that the McKenzie exercise program is the correct one for you.

The centralization of pain is the single most important guide you have in determining which exercises are correct for your problem. The phenomenon of centralization of pain has now been scientifically validated. Several studies in the United States have demonstrated that if your pain centralizes when you perform the exercises, your chances of rapid and complete recovery are *excellent.*

On the other hand, *avoid activities or positions that cause the pain to "peripheralize"—to move away from the center of the lower back or from the lower back entirely. Also avoid activities and positions that increase any pain in the buttock or leg.*

When first doing the exercises, be cautious and don't hurry. If your lower back pain is of such intensity that you can move around only with difficulty and cannot find a position in which to lie comfortably in bed, you should approach the exercises in an especially cautious and unhurried manner.

When you begin any of the exercises, you may at first experience an increase in pain. *This initial increase of pain is common and can be expected.* As you continue to practice, the pain should quickly diminish, at least to the level you experienced before beginning the exercises. *The reduction of pain, at*

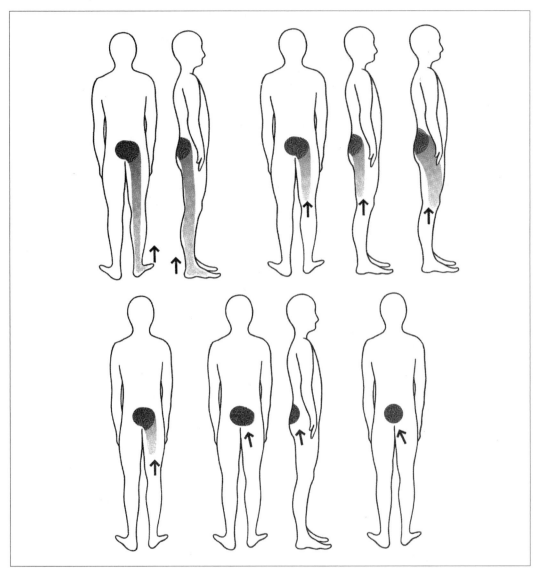

Figure 5.1: The progressive centralization of pain as a result of the McKenzie exercise program

least to the original level, usually occurs during the first exercise session. In the first exercise session or a later one, the reduction of pain should be followed by centralization of pain.

Once the pain no longer spreads outward and instead is felt only at the midline, the intensity of pain will decrease rapidly over a period of two to three days. In one to four weeks, your pain should disappear entirely.

If, however, following an initial increase in pain, the pain continues to increase or spreads to places farther away from the spine, immediately stop exercising. Seek advice from a health professional. In other words, do not continue with any of the exercises if your symptoms are much worse immediately after exercising and remain throughout the day. Also stop the exercises if, during exercise, you experience symptoms in the leg below the knee for the first time or if you experience a worsening in symptoms that you already had below the knee.

If your symptoms have been present more or less continuously for many weeks or months, you should not expect to be pain free in two or three days. The response will be slower than if your symptoms were recent, but if you are doing the correct exercises, it will usually be only a week before improvement begins. If you are lucky, it will be faster than that.

When beginning this exercise program, you should stop any other exercises that you may have been shown by a health professional. You should also temporarily stop any workouts or sports activities. If you want to continue with exercises other than those described in this book, you should wait until your pain has completely subsided. If you are intent on returning to sports before your pain has subsided, you must nonetheless avoid all contact sports. As for noncontact sports, you can gently attempt a return to them; if, after a short trial, your pain is worse, you must discontinue even noncontact sports until your pain has completely subsided.

Once you have started this exercise program, new pains may develop, because you are performing movements your body is not used to. But, provided you continue with the exercises, these pains will wear off in a few days. I always suspect that if my patients do not complain of new pains, they have not been exercising adequately or they have not been putting enough effort into correcting their posture. Both new exercises and new postures *should* cause temporary new pains.

I cannot overstress the importance of doing the exercises precisely as they are described in this book. That is, it is important to do each exercise exactly as it is described and to do the exercises in the order that is set out in this book. The failure to heed even one sentence in the description of an exercise can keep the exercise from being effective. Don't figure that you can save time by glancing at the instructions for a particular exercise or by trying to learn an exercise just by looking at the photographs that accompany it. In this way you may save a minute or two, but slow your recovery by weeks—not a good bargain.

Similarly, don't skimp. Generally, the exercises should be done six to eight times a day. If you do them once or twice a day, you may gain some benefit, but not nearly what you would gain if you did them as often as prescribed.

RESEARCH SUPPORTS THE METHOD

Decades' worth of clinical experience and research lie behind these exercises: how to do them, in what order to do them, how often to do them.

The findings presented in Adelaide, Australia, in April 2000 are as important as any research ever done on the McKenzie Method. Presented to the International Society for the Study of the Lumbar Spine, the study involved patients who had suffered from back pain for an average of 10.4 years. They had seen an average of 2.5 health care providers before entering the study.

As an abstract of the study says, this was "a dissertation-based investigation of the impact of reading a specific booklet on the LBP [low back pain] and self-treatment behaviour of volunteer chronic symptomatic subjects." These subjects were not treated by doctors, physical therapists, or anybody else. They were treated only by themselves, and the only information they had was a "booklet." In fact, the "booklet" was a detailed description of the McKenzie Method, demonstrating the exercises and posture control found in the book you are reading.

One week after reading the booklet, 86 percent of the study participants were confident they could treat their own pain effectively. Eighty-five percent said they would use the booklet as a reference and would also use it to "self-treat" in the event of an acute episode and to prevent pain in the future.

Fifty-two percent reported reduced pain in the first week. Once the subjects had used the booklet for nine months, 87 percent were still regularly using the exercises in the booklet and 91 percent were still focusing on good posture.

Most important, at nine months, 82 percent had less back pain and 60 percent were completely free of pain. Of those who used the booklet, 95 percent said it was responsible for their improvement.

At the beginning of the study, subjects reported pain that averaged 1.3 on a scale of 4. At nine months, subjects reported pain that averaged only 0.44 on the same scale.

At the start, subjects reported an average of 4.1 episodes of back pain per year. After reading the booklet, they averaged just 1.0 episode per year. (B. Undermann et al., 2000, "Can an Educational Booklet Change Behavior and Pain in Chronic Low Back Patients?" International Society for the Study of the Lumbar Spine, Adelaide, Australia.)

These subjects did well because they carefully followed the instructions in the booklet. Similarly, you will do well if you carefully follow the instructions in this book. I want you to benefit as much as possible from the exercises and posture control. Don't get in the way of your own recovery!

BACK EXERCISE 1

Lying Facedown

This is the first McKenzie exercise for the *lower back*. Again, if you are a *neck* patient, you will find the McKenzie exercises for the neck in Chapter 12. Shoulder sufferers will find relief in the exercises that may be found in Chapter 21. This exercise is not suitable for pregnant patients.

An exercise session is a series of repetitions of one or more exercises. Until you can do one or more of the other McKenzie back exercises without acute pain, each time you exercise you must begin with Back Exercise 1, followed by Back Exercise 2.

Lie facedown with your arms next to your body. Your arms should be straight but relaxed. Your head should be turned to one side. (See Fig. 5.2.) Stay in this position, then take a few deep breaths, and then relax completely for two or three minutes. You must make a conscious effort to remove all tension from the muscles in your lower back, hips, and legs: without this complete relaxation, there is no chance of eliminating any distortion that may be present in the joints.

Back Exercise 1 is used mainly in the treatment of acute back pain (back pain that has begun recently and is sharp, as opposed to chronic back pain,

Figure 5.2: Lie facedown with your arms next to your body and your head turned to one side.

which has gone on for a long time and is rather a dull ache). In fact, Exercise 1 is one of the McKenzie Method's *first-aid exercises.* This exercise should be done once at the beginning of each exercise session. Ordinarily, you should do this exercise once per session, but you may feel free to do it more often than that. The exercise sessions should be spread evenly throughout the day, for a total of six to eight times. This means that you should repeat the sessions about every two hours. In addition, you should lie facedown whenever you are resting.

Back Exercise 1 is performed in preparation for Exercise 2.

BACK EXERCISE 2

Lying Facedown in Extension

Back Exercise 2 must be done only after Exercise 1 has been completed. Remain facedown (Fig. 5.3a), in the same position you used in Exercise 1. This too is an exercise that is not safe for patients who are pregnant.

Now place your elbows under your shoulders so that you lean on your forearms (Fig. 5.3b). During this exercise (as with Exercise 1), begin by taking a few deep breaths and then allowing the muscles in the lower back, hips, and legs to relax completely. Remain in this position for two to three minutes.

Exercise 2 is used mainly in the treatment of acute lower back pain and, like Exercise 1, is one of the *first-aid exercises.* It is also of great benefit for patients with chronic or recurrent problems. Exercise 2 should be done once per exercise session. As with Exercise 1, the sessions should be repeated about every two hours.

If you experience acute, increasing pain when you attempt this exercise, move your elbows farther away from your body (to the sides), so that your top half is lowered to a point at which your pain is tolerable. Alternatively, you can place a pillow under your chest for a few moments until the pain decreases.

If these efforts are not helpful, there are certain measures you must take before you can continue exercising. These are discussed in Chapter 6, under the heading "When You Get No Response or Benefit." Go to that section now.

This exercise is performed in preparation for Back Exercise 3.

Figure 5.3a: Remain facedown.

Figure 5.3b: Place your elbows under your shoulders so that you lean on your forearms.

BACK EXERCISE 3

Extension in Lying

Before doing this exercise for the first time, start your exercise session with Back Exercise 1, followed by Exercise 2. If you are pregnant, do not attempt this exercise.

Remain facedown, but with your head forward rather than to the side (Fig. 5.4a). Place your hands under your shoulders in the position you would use for a push-up (Fig. 5.4b). Now you are ready to commence Back Exercise 3.

CASE HISTORY: ENGINEERING HER OWN RECOVERY

Helen is a civil engineer, age fifty-two, and lives in upstate New York. She had lower back pain for eight years. The pain was worse when she sat or bent over. She got some relief simply by using a lumbar roll, by walking, and by standing.

Before starting the McKenzie program, Helen had seen numerous physical therapists and a chiropractor, attended a "back school," and endured two epidural injections for pain. A doctor had diagnosed degenerative disc disease.

Helen used Back Exercise 3, Extension in Lying. This led to increased extension range without any worsening of pain. Five days after starting the program, her lower back pain had decreased. Helen continued with Exercise 3, making a special effort to "sag" as much as possible. Sagging caused pain at the end of her range of motion, but the pain did not remain when she left the extreme sag position.

Two days later Helen had full range of motion. She began the slouch-overcorrect technique without any pain and was able to do Back Exercise 4, Extension in Standing, fully extended.

Five days later, she progressed to Back Exercise 5, Flexion in Lying.

Seventeen days later, Helen had no symptoms at all. Even two weeks after starting, Helen had no pain and no limitation in range of motion. Seventeen days after starting, she had no symptoms at all.

Straighten your elbows and push the top half of your body—the part from the pelvis on up—up as far as pain permits (Fig. 5.4c). As you do this, it is important that you completely relax the pelvis, hips, and legs. *Keep your pelvis, hips, and legs hanging limp and allow your back to sag.* Your pelvis will naturally move downward.

Once you have maintained this position for a second or two, lower yourself to the starting position. Each time you repeat the cycle of movements in this exercise, try to raise your upper body a little higher, so that by the last repetition of this exercise within a session your back is extended as much as possible and your arms are as straight as possible with your elbows locked (Fig. 5.4d).

Each time you straighten your arms, remember to hold the sag for a second or two, because this is a key part of the exercise. If you feel your pain is decreasing or centralizing (or both), you may maintain the sag for longer than one or two seconds.

As with all other McKenzie Method back, neck, and shoulder exercises involving multiple movements, remember to slowly think or say the words "pressure on, pressure off" as you do the exercise. This helps you to hold each position just long enough and establishes a rhythm in which to do the exercise.

Back Exercise 3 is the most useful and effective first-aid procedure in the treatment of acute lower back pain. The exercise can also be used to treat stiffness of the lower back and to prevent lower back pain from recurring once you have fully recovered. When used in the treatment of either pain or stiffness, the exercise should be performed ten times per session. Again, exercise sessions should be spread evenly six to eight times throughout the day.

Should you not respond to Back Exercise 3 or should you have increasing pain when you attempt this exercise, there are certain measures you must take before you can continue exercising. These are discussed in Chapter 6, under the heading "When You Get No Response or Benefit." Go to that section now.

Remember that if your pain has *centralized*, it may have *increased* in the middle of your back after it has disappeared from one side or from your leg. This does *not* indicate that you are not responding or benefiting. In fact, this is a good response, and you should continue with the exercises. If the pain has

Figure 5.4a: Remain facedown.

Figure 5.4b: Place your hands under your shoulders in the push-up position.

Figure 5.4c: Straighten your elbows and push the top half of your body up as far as pain permits.

Figure 5.4d: At the end of your exercise, your back is extended as much as possible and your arms are as straight as possible.

increased but has centralized, you need not read "When You Get No Response or Benefit."

BACK EXERCISE 4

Extension in Standing

Stand upright, with your feet slightly apart. Place your hands in the small of your back with the fingers pointing backward (Figs. 5.5a and 5.5b). You are now ready to begin Back Exercise 4. But there is one group who must not try this exercise: patients who are pregnant.

Bend your trunk backward at the waist *as far as you can*, using your hands as a fulcrum (Figs. 5.5c and 5.5d). As you do this, it is important that you *keep your knees straight*. Once you have maintained this position for a second or two, return to the starting position. Each time you repeat the cycle of movements in this exercise, try to bend backward a little farther so that by the last repetition your back is extended as far as possible.

When you are in acute pain, Back Exercise 4 may replace Exercise 3 if circumstances prevent you from exercising in the lying position. Nevertheless, this exercise is not as effective as Exercise 3. In the event that you replace Exercise 3 with Exercise 4, do Exercise 4 as often as you would have done Exercise 3; that is, ten times per session, six to eight sessions a day.

Once you are fully recovered and no longer have lower back pain, Back Exercise 4 is *your main tool in the prevention of further lower back problems*. As a preventive measure, repeat Exercise 4 every once in a while whenever you find yourself working in a forward-bent position. Perform the exercise *before* the pain appears.

One of the beauties of Exercise 4 is that it can be done without lying down. Therefore, in public or business settings, you can do this exercise more easily than you can perform those that require you to lie down. Still, you should make every effort to find a way to do the lying-down exercises approximately every two hours.

Figure 5.5a: Stand upright, with your feet slightly apart. Place your hands in the small of your back with your fingers pointing backward.

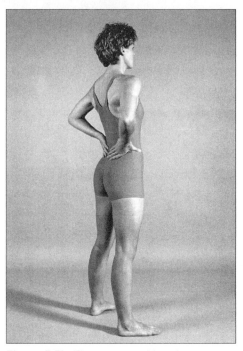

Figure 5.5b: The same position, from a different perspective

Figure 5.5c: Bend your trunk backward at the waist as far as you can, using your hands as a fulcrum.

Figure 5.5d: The same position, from a different perspective

BACK EXERCISE 5

Flexion in Lying

Although some who have heard of the McKenzie Method believe it involves extension and nothing but extension, this is not the case. I have found that for many patients, certain flexion exercises can also be helpful. But especially with the flexion exercises, timing is the key to success. (See later in this chapter; also see Chapter 6, "When to Do the Back Exercises.")

Lie on your back with your knees bent and your feet flat on the floor or bed (Fig. 5.6a). You are now ready to begin Back Exercise 5.

> **NOTE:** The following two motions (Figs. 5.6b and 5.6c) should be performed with extra caution.

Bring both knees up toward your chest (Fig. 5.6b). Place both hands around your knees and gently but firmly pull your knees as close to your chest as pain permits (Fig. 5.6c). Once you have maintained this position for a second or two, lower the legs and return to the starting position. It is important that you *do not raise your head* as you perform this exercise. It is also important that you *do not straighten your legs as you lower them.*

Each time you repeat the cycle of movements in this exercise, try to pull your knees a little closer to the chest, so that by the last repetition of this exercise you have flexed your back as much as possible.

Figure 5.6a: Lie on your back with your knees bent and your feet flat on the floor or bed.

Figure 5.6b: Bring both knees up toward your chest.

Figure 5.6c: Place both hands around your knees and gently but firmly pull your knees as close to your chest as pain permits.

Juan is sixty-four and manages a plant nursery. He lives in New Jersey. Before beginning the McKenzie program, he had suffered from central lower back pain for three weeks. This appeared after a week during which an employee was out sick and Juan did a lot of stooping as he performed the tasks of the employee. The pain spread to his right calf, and his doctor diagnosed him as having sciatica.

Any activity made his symptoms worse, to the point that he had to lie down to get relief. These activities included sitting, standing, and walking. A non-McKenzie physical therapist had instructed Juan to do exercises that involved lumbar flexion, and these only made his pain more intense.

Juan's posture, though not perfect, was fairly erect, and his range of motion was normal for his age. Though lumbar flexion movements had worsened his pain, he found that the opposite, McKenzie Back Exercise 3, Extension in Lying, eliminated it. He also found it helpful to improve his posture by using the slouch-overcorrect method and a lumbar roll.

With the McKenzie program, Juan remained pain free even during the activities that previously had caused him symptoms.

You can use this exercise to treat stiffness in the lower back that may have developed since your injury began. While damaged tissues may now have healed, they may also have shortened and become less flexible. It is now necessary to restore their elasticity and full function by performing flexion exercises.

Begin these exercises with caution. Do only five or six repetitions per session, and repeat the sessions three or four times a day. As you have probably realized, once your knees are bent in this exercise, you have eliminated the lordosis. Therefore, in order to correct any distortion that may result, *this and all other flexion exercises (that is, Back Exercises 5, 6, and 7) must always be followed immediately by a session of Exercise 3, Extension in Lying.*

BACK EXERCISE 6

Flexion in Sitting

Begin doing Back Exercise 6 only after you have completed one week of Exercise 5, whether or not Exercise 5 has been successful in reducing your pain or stiffness.

Sit on the edge of a steady chair. Your knees and feet should be well apart. Rest your hands on your legs (Fig. 5.7a). Now you are ready to begin Exercise 6.

Bend your trunk forward and grasp your ankles or touch the floor with your hands (Fig. 5.7b). Return immediately to the starting position. Each time you repeat the cycle of movements in this exercise, try to bend down a little farther so that by the last repetition of this exercise you have flexed your back as much as possible and your head is as close as possible to the floor.

This exercise can be made more effective by holding on to your ankles with your hands and pulling yourself down farther (Figs. 5.7c and 5.7d).

Figure 5.7a: Sit on the edge of a steady chair with your knees and feet well apart and rest your hands on your legs.

Figure 5.7b: Bend your trunk forward and grasp your ankles or touch the floor with your hands.

Figure 5.7c: Hold on to your ankles and pull yourself down farther.

Figure 5.7d: Or even farther

You must do only five or six repetitions of Exercise 6 per session. Sessions are to be repeated three to four times a day. *Back Exercise 6 must always be followed immediately by a session of Exercise 3, Extension in Lying.*

BACK EXERCISE 7

Flexion in Standing

Begin doing Back Exercise 7 only after you have completed two weeks of Exercise 6, whether or not Exercise 6 has been successful in reducing your pain or stiffness.

Stand upright, with your feet well apart. Allow your arms to hang loosely by your sides (Fig. 5.8a). You are now ready to begin Exercise 7.

Bend forward and run your fingers down your legs as far as you can

Figure 5.8a: Stand upright with your feet well apart and allow your arms to hang loosely by your side.

Figure 5.8b: Bend forward and run your fingers down your legs as far as you can comfortably reach.

comfortably reach (Fig. 5.8b). Return immediately to the upright standing position. Each time you repeat the cycle of movements in this exercise, try to bend down a little farther so that by the last repetition of this exercise within a session you have flexed your back as much as possible and your fingertips are as close as possible to the floor.

You must do only five or six repetitions of Exercise 7 per session. Sessions are to be repeated once or twice a day. *Back Exercise 7 must always be followed immediately by a session of Exercise 3, Extension in Lying.*

For three months after you have become pain free, Exercise 7 must never be performed in the first four hours of your day.

6 WHEN TO DO THE BACK EXERCISES

You should seek advice from your doctor if your back pain is of such severity that it is impossible to perform these exercises (or other exercises in this book) or your pain is becoming intolerable.

YOU PROBABLY HAVE EXPERIENCED SEVERAL ACUTE OR SEVERE EPIsodes of back pain in the past. You probably already know that the pain will decrease in time. Still, you may never have been completely free of pain. (Chronic patients can find special hope in the recent research, mentioned in Chapter 5, that studied people who had had back pain for an average of ten years. After nine months using the McKenzie exercise program, 60 percent were pain free, and an additional 22 percent had less pain.) What can you do to speed your recovery from a particular episode or rid yourself of chronic pain?

This chapter is aimed at assisting you to make a more rapid recovery than you have before. In learning how to accelerate your recovery, you will at the same time learn steps you must take in the future if trouble strikes again. And yes, it can happen again. Because once you feel good, you, like all others with the same problem, will tend to forget the precautions you should take. The main thing is to learn how the movements described in this chapter affect your particular back problem.

WHEN YOU ARE IN SIGNIFICANT PAIN

A severe attack of lower back pain may involve pain that is felt at all times regardless of the position you adopt or the movements you perform. This pain is made much worse by sitting or by arising from a sitting position and bending forward. If the pain is also much worse when you attempt to stand up or walk, and if you are unable to straighten up fully, it may not be possible for you to function, and bed rest is your only alternative.

Recent research tells us that bed rest is not the best option for the treatment of acute and severe back pain and should be used for no more than two days. Those involved in that research, however, may alter their view if they ever personally experience a severe bout of back pain.

In my experience, there are many patients in severe pain who require longer than two days of bed rest before it is possible for them to walk. Nevertheless, early exercise and other movement is preferred for those forced to seek bed rest, and a determined effort to stand upright should be attempted at least once each day.

You may begin the exercise program during your period of bed rest, provided you can lie facedown for short periods. Perform Back Exercises 1 through 3: Lying Facedown, Lying Facedown in Extension, and Extension in Lying (Figs. 6.1a–c). *These exercises are first aid for lower back pain.* Immediately following the exercises, roll onto your back and insert the lumbar roll described in Chapter 4, under the heading "Correcting the Surface for Lying Down." This will maintain your back in the correct position during the period of bed rest.

If your back pain is so severe that it is impossible for you to perform any of the exercises or if your pain is becoming intolerable, seek advice from your family physician. Certain over-the-counter (OTC) medications, such as aspirin and other nonsteroidal anti-inflammatory drugs (NSAIDs), one of the best known of which is ibuprofen (found under brand names such as Advil and also available as a less expensive generic drug), may be necessary to provide some relief from pain. Aspirin and other OTC NSAIDs have been found to be highly effective for reducing acute back pain and have fewer side effects than some common prescription drugs. Both aspirin and other NSAIDs have been recommended by the U.S. government's Agency for Health Care Policy and Research (now the Agency for Healthcare Research and Quality).

Figure 6.1a: Exercise 1

Figure 6.1b: Exercise 2

Figure 6.1c: Exercise 3

Likewise, if your pain is not severe enough to force you to rest in bed, and you are able to continue with some of your daily activities in spite of your pain, perform Back Exercises 1 through 3: Lying Facedown, Lying Facedown in Extension, and Extension in Lying.

The aim in performing Exercises 1 through 3 is to restore the lordosis to the fullest possible extent; then you must maintain it by paying careful attention, at all times during the first week, to both posture and movements. Avoid rounded postures that occur when bending or sitting slouched, and in fact sit as little as possible. Therefore, by avoiding flexion, you remove the cause of any further distortion within the joint, and you allow healing to occur. (Remember the example of bending the finger? And the slippery bar of soap?)

When you begin Exercise 3, at first you may experience an increase in pain in the lower back. But as you repeat the exercise, the pain should gradually decrease so that there is significant improvement within a few sessions. The pain may also become more localized in the center of the back (this is the process of centralization, discussed in the previous chapter). This is desirable, as is any movement of pain from the legs and buttocks toward the middle of the back. In time, the pain should disappear and be replaced by a feeling of strain or stiffness, which is more tolerable.

If your pain does not centralize, decrease, or otherwise improve with these exercises, please immediately read "When You Get No Response or Benefit" later in this chapter.

As soon as you feel considerably better and no longer have constant pain— perhaps a day or two after you have begun exercising—*you may stop Back Exercises 1 and 2,* but you must continue Exercise 3 and you must add Exercise 4, Extension in Standing. At about this time you must slowly introduce the postural slouch-overcorrect procedure discussed in Chapter 4, because you must now learn to sit correctly and maintain the lordosis just short of its maximum. As a rule, the pain will decrease as the lordosis increases, and you will have no pain at all once you maintain the correct sitting posture. Pain will readily recur if you forget your posture and lose that vital hollow in your lower back. Exercise 4 should be done whenever circumstances keep you from performing Exercise 3: at regular intervals during sitting and working in a stooped position, and before and after lifting as well as during repeated lifting. The slouch-overcorrect procedure must be done two or three times per day until you are familiar with the correct sitting posture.

Once you no longer have acute pain, continue the exercise program as outlined next.

WHEN ACUTE PAIN HAS SUBSIDED

For the past few days you have been doing Back Exercises 1 to 4 and have been maintaining a lordosis at all times. Once the distortion in the joints has decreased and any damaged tissue has healed, you will need to restore your flexibility and recover your normal function. Flexibility is best achieved by doing flexion exercises, which must be performed in such a way that no further damage or tearing occurs within soft tissues that have recently healed. The risks of further damage are much less when the lower back is rounded in the lying position than when it is in the standing position. Therefore you must now do Back Exercise 5, Flexion in Lying (Fig. 6.2a)—and follow each session with Exercise 3 (Fig. 6.2b).

You should begin Flexion in Lying when you have mostly recovered from an acute episode of lower back pain and have had long pain-free periods for two to three weeks, even though you may still feel stiffness when you bend forward. Exercise 5 may also be necessary if you have improved significantly with Exercises 1 through 4 but after two or three weeks still experience a small amount of pain at the center of your back, pain that seems like it will not disappear.

Figure 6.2a: Exercise 5, to be followed by . . .

Figure 6.2b: . . . Exercise 3

It is not uncommon for some central, midline, lower back pain to occur when you start Back Exercise 5. An initial pain that wears off gradually with repetition of the exercise is acceptable; it means that shortened structures are being stretched effectively. *If Exercise 5 causes pain that increases with each repetition, stop.* In this case, it is probably too soon to start flexion and you should wait and try it in another week or two.

When you can touch your chest with your knees easily and without discomfort, you have regained full movement. You may now stop Back Exercise 5 and begin Exercise 6 (Fig. 6.3). After two to three weeks, Exercise 6 should cause no tightness or discomfort, and once you have reached this point, you may add Exercise 7 to your program (Fig. 6.4).

NOTE: Back Exercises 5, 6, and 7 should always be followed immediately by Exercise 3, Extension in Lying (Fig. 6.2b). In this way, you can rectify any distortion that could develop from Exercises 5, 6, or 7.

Back Exercise 7 should be carried out at the end of the day once or twice a week to ensure that all the soft tissues in the back remain able to flex. After completing Exercises 5 and 7, follow the guidelines given to prevent recurrence of lower back problems and continue with the exercise program. This is discussed further in the next section.

Figure 6.3: Exercise 6

Figure 6.4: Exercise 7

WHEN YOU HAVE NO PAIN OR STIFFNESS

Many people with lower back problems have long spells in which they experience little or no pain. If, in the past or recently, you have had one or more episodes of lower back pain, start or continue the exercise program even though you may be pain free at the moment. In this situation it is not necessary to do all the exercises, nor is it necessary to exercise every two hours.

To prevent recurrence of lower back problems:

1. Perform Back Exercise 3, Extension in Lying, on a regular basis, preferably in the morning and evening.
2. Perform Back Exercise 4, Extension in Standing, at regular intervals whenever you must sit or bend forward for long periods. Also do Exercise 4 before and after heavy lifting and during repeated lifting, as well as whenever you feel minor strain developing in your lower back.
3. Practice the slouch-overcorrect procedure (see Chapter 4) whenever you are becoming careless about the correct sitting posture.
4. Perform Back Exercise 7 once or twice a week to remain fully flexible.
5. Always use a lumbar roll in chairs that do not provide adequate support.

Continue these exercises and adopt them as a regular part of your life. It is essential, however, that you do them *before the onset of pain*. Even more important than exercising, you must watch your posture at all times and never again let postural stresses become the cause of

Figure 6.5: Lie facedown.

lower back problems. The best exercises will have little or no effect if you constantly fall back into poor posture.

Therefore, you should exercise in the manner described above for the rest of your life, but you *must* develop and maintain good postural habits. Remember, if you lose the lordosis for long periods at a time, you risk the recurrence of lower back pain.

Because it takes only one minute to perform one session of Back Exercise 3 and two minutes to complete one session of the slouch-overcorrect procedure, lack of time should never be used as an excuse for not doing these exercises.

WHEN YOU GET NO RESPONSE OR BENEFIT

After exercising without any relief or benefit for three or four days, you may conclude that the back exercises as performed are ineffective. But there are two main situations that can lead to an apparent lack of response or benefit from the exercises presented in this book, and both are rectifiable.

People whose pain is felt only to one side of the spine, or whose pain is felt much more to one side than the other, may experience a lack of response to these exercises. If your pain during the course of the day is felt only to one side, or more to one side than the other, or if you feel pain more to one side as you perform Back Exercises 1, 2, or 3, you may need to modify your body position before you begin these exercises.

Figure 6.6a–b: Move your hips away from the pain.

Here is how to modify your body position:

1. Position yourself to perform Back Exercise 1 and allow yourself to relax for a few minutes (Fig. 6.5).
2. Remain facedown, then shift your hips away from the painful side. That is, if your pain usually is more on the right side, you must move your hips

Figure 6.7a–b: With hips off-center, lean on elbows.

three or four inches to the left and once more completely relax for a few minutes (Figs. 6.6a and 6.6b).

3. While allowing the hips to remain off center, lean on the elbows as described in Back Exercise 2 and relax for an additional three or four minutes (Figs. 6.7a and 6.7b).

You are now ready to begin Back Exercise 3. With your hips still off center, complete one session of Exercise 3 (Figs. 6.8a and 6.8b) and then relax once more. You may need to repeat the exercise several times, but before beginning each session of ten, ensure that your hips are still off center: remember, away from the painful side. Even with your hips in the off-center position, try in each repetition to move higher and higher. Reach the maximum amount of extension possible, at which point your arms should be completely straight.

For the next three or four days, continue to perform Back Exercises 1, 2, and 3 from the modified starting position described in the three steps above. The frequency of the exercises and the number of sessions per day should be the same as recommended in the section titled "When You Are in Significant Pain," at the beginning of this chapter.

After a few days of practice, you may notice that the pain is distributed more evenly across the back or has centralized. Once this occurs, you may stop shifting the hips before exercising and continue exercises as recommended

Figure 6.8a–b: With hips off center, you are ready to begin Exercise 3.

earlier, under "When You Are in Significant Pain." Occasionally, shifting the hips away from the painful side is sufficient to stop the pain completely.

The second situation that may impede a person's response is when Back Exercise 3 is done without the pelvis remaining more or less immobilized in a low position. In this case, Exercise 3 occasionally gives benefit for only a few hours, and then the pain returns.

The effectiveness of Exercise 3 can be improved greatly by holding the pelvis down. There are two main ways to do this. Another person can place pressure on your lower back. Or you can construct a simple device for keeping your pelvis in place: you can use an ironing board and either a seat belt or a strong leather belt or strap. Place the belt or strap around the ironing board and your waistline and proceed with Exercise 3 (Fig. 6.9). The added pressure frequently makes the difference.

WHEN YOU HAVE A RECURRENCE

Regardless of what you are doing or where you are, at the first sign of recurrence of lower back pain you must take action. That is, you must immediately start the exercises that previously led to recovery, and you must follow the

Figure 6.9: Added pressure

instructions given to relieve acute pain. You must at once begin Back Exercise 4, Extension in Standing. If this does not eliminate your pain *within minutes*, you must quickly introduce Exercise 3, Extension in Lying. *The immediate use of Exercise 3 very often can prevent the onset of a disabling attack of lower back pain.* If your pain is already too acute to tolerate these exercises, begin with Exercises 1 and 2, Lying Facedown and Lying Facedown in Extension.

Finally, if you have symptoms on one side that do not centralize as a result of the exercises just recommended, shift your hips away from the painful side before beginning the exercises. Further, hold your hips in the off-center position while you exercise. In addition to the exercises, you must pay extra attention to your posture and maintain the lordosis as much as possible.

If your new episode of lower back pain seems to be different from those you have experienced on other occasions, and if your pain persists despite the fact that you have closely followed the instructions in this book, seek advice from a health professional, ideally a member or associate of the McKenzie Institute.

To obtain the names of credentialed members and associates of the McKenzie Institute, see Appendix A at the back of this book.

7 INSTRUCTIONS FOR PEOPLE WITH ACUTE LOWER BACK PAIN

IMMEDIATELY BEGIN THE SELF-TREATMENT EXERCISES

The simple rule is that if bending forward has caused overstretching, bending backward should rectify this problem and reduce any resultant distortion in the spinal discs. You must restore the lordosis slowly and with caution, never quickly or with jerky movements. You must allow some time for the distorted joint to regain its normal shape and position. A sudden or violent movement may retard this process, increase the strain in and around the affected joint, and thereby result in an increase of lower back pain.

Whenever you are not certain that you recall precisely how to do the exercises, go back to their descriptions in this book and read each line of any exercise you do not recall in detail. Reviewing the exercises is a small price to pay for feeling better. A reminder of Exercises 1, 2, and 3 is found in the photographs at the end of this chapter (Figs. 7.1a–c).

Remember, when you begin the exercises, some increase of midline lower back pain can be expected. Some exercises will be effective only when you actually move into the pain while exercising. You should feel some pain when doing these exercises, but you should never have an increase in pain that lasts into the following day.

When in acute pain, you must, in addition to performing these exercises, make certain adjustments in your daily activities. These adjustments form a very important aspect of self-treatment. If you do not follow the instructions given below, you will unnecessarily delay the healing process. *Following the instructions is entirely your responsibility.*

Maintain your lumbar lordosis at all times. Slouched sitting and bending forward, as when touching the toes, will only increase the pressure in the joints, stretch and weaken the supporting structures, and lead to further damage in the lower back. If you slouch, you will have discomfort and pain. *Good posture is the key to spinal comfort.*

Sit as little as possible, and even then only for short periods. If you must sit, choose a firm, high chair with a straight back, make sure you have an adequate lordosis, and use a lumbar roll to support the lower back. Avoid sitting on a low, soft couch with your legs straight out in front; also avoid sitting up in bed or the bath; all these situations force you to lose the lordosis.

When getting up from the sitting position, try to maintain the lordosis: move to the front of the seat (or carefully rotate to the exit edge of a seat in a car), stand up by straightening the legs, and avoid bending forward at the waist.

If you have a car, drive it as little as possible. It is better to be a passenger than to be the driver. Whether you are the driver or a passenger, be sure to bring along your lumbar roll. If you must be the driver, your seat should be far enough back from the steering wheel to allow you to drive with your arms relatively straight. With the arms straight, your upper body is held back and you are prevented from slouching; this allows full benefit to be obtained from the lumbar roll.

Avoid activities that require bending forward or stooping. Many activities can be modified enough that you can maintain your lordosis. To the surprise of some, it is possible to maintain the correct standing posture while vacuuming; it is also possible to maintain a correct lordosis when getting down on "all fours" when gardening or making a bed.

If you have acute lower back pain, you should not lift at all. If you must lift, avoid objects that are awkward to handle or heavier than thirty pounds (about fifteen kilograms). At all times you must use the correct lifting technique.

If you are uncomfortable while sleeping or attempting to sleep, you may benefit from a supportive roll around your waist. For most people, the mattress should not be too hard but should be well supported by a firm base. If your bed sags, slats or a sheet of plywood (a "bed board") between mattress and base will straighten it; as an alternative, you can place the mattress on the floor.

CASE HISTORY: HOLLYWOOD BARBARA

Barbara is a Hollywood entertainment executive specializing in the production of documentaries. She works long hours at her desk and also drives to many meetings, screenings, and other events. At age fifty-two, after many years of the same habits, she developed lower back pain that sometimes was sharp. She adapted her chair at work by using a lumbar roll, and after a while rarely had pain at the office.

Her main complaint then became pain while in the car. She didn't have much trouble while driving, but had almost excruciating pain when exiting the vehicle. She was confused about the cause, thinking it must be the exiting rather than the driving.

Her friend Bill sent her the instructions for my exercises. A busy woman who rarely initiates calls, she nevertheless called Bill the day after receiving the exercises. "I'm a lot better!" she exclaimed in relief and surprise. She had been helped by the McKenzie exercises (especially Back Exercise 3, Extension in Lying). But she also had benefited from the discussion of the fact that posture is the key to most back pain. She therefore began to use a lumbar roll in the car even though driving rarely was accompanied by pain. The roll helped.

She did best, however, when she paid special attention to the McKenzie Method's advice on how to maintain the lower back lordosis even as one moves from a sitting position to a standing position. In summary, the method says to move to the front of a regular chair or to the exit side of a car seat, then to stand up by straightening the legs, while taking care not to bend forward at the waist. Similarly, when you have been lying down and you want to get up, keep your back in lordosis: turn on one side, pull both knees up, drop your feet over the edge of the bed, raise yourself to the sitting position by pushing your upper body up with your hands, and avoid bending forward at the waist.

With the combination of lumbar rolls at the office and in the car, the exercises, and the technique for getting out of a sitting posture, Barbara became almost entirely pain free.

Figure 7.1a: Exercise 1

Figuere 7.1b: Exercise 2

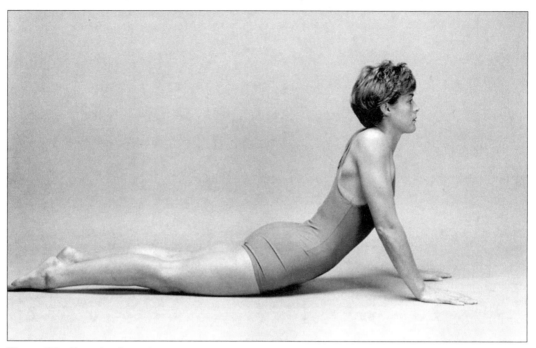

Figure 7.1c: Exercise 3

Avoid coughing and sneezing while you are sitting or bending forward. If you must cough or sneeze, stand and bend backward.

Avoid those positions and movements that caused your problems in the first place.

Allow some time for healing to take place.

(In the event that you have a sudden onset of acute lower back pain and need a super quick summary of what to do, consult Chapter 15, "Panic Pages for the Back.")

8 SPECIAL BACK SITUATIONS

TREATMENT BY REPEX

Although the system of self-treatment that I have developed is effective for a very high percentage of patients, the success of the method is sometimes limited because of various factors that may prevent the patient from performing the required movements.

Fatigue is probably the limiting factor that patients encounter most commonly. They find they are unable to continue exercising because their arms have become too tired. This is particularly frustrating for the patient whose pain is improving with the exercises but who cannot continue them because of fatigue.

Some patients are unable to relax enough when they perform the push-up exercise (Back Exercise 3). For the exercise to be effective, it is vital that your lower back be relaxed.

Some patients, especially the elderly, have shoulder, elbow, or wrist problems that keep them from performing the key exercises.

Patients with certain disorders have such restricted movements that the exercises in this book are impossible to perform.

But all is not lost!

To overcome these difficulties, in 1986 I engaged an engineer to develop a machine to provide controlled doses of specific repeated movements for the lower back.

The machine is named REPEX. It can continuously move the lower back many hundreds of times if necessary, without the patient having to exert himself or herself at all. And that's why REPEX has the name it does: it stands for *repeated end-range passive exercise*. ("End-range" refers to the end of a patient's range of movement.)

The REPEX machine provides a type of treatment known as CPM, or continuous passive motion. Before REPEX came along, CPM had been found to provide better-quality healing and more rapid recovery when applied to other injured joints of the body. REPEX is the first machine to provide CPM for lower back disorders.

If you have not already resolved your back problem with the McKenzie Method as described in this book, it may well be that the REPEX can assist you further. It is particularly likely that REPEX can help with your problem *if you get relief after each session of exercise but the relief does not last*. In this case, it may well be that an increased number of movements—possible with REPEX—may be all that is required to give you lasting relief.

Treatment by REPEX requires the expertise of a specialist. This treatment is available only through credentialed members and associates of the McKenzie Institute.

To obtain the names of credentialed members and associates of the McKenzie Institute, see Appendix A of this book.

REPEX is available from Hill Laboratories Company, Frazer, Pennsylvania: www.hilllabs.com.

LOWER BACK PAIN IN PREGNANCY

Both during and after pregnancy, women are subjected to altered mechanical stresses that affect the lower back and frequently result in lower back problems. As the new infant develops in the mother's womb, two simple changes occur that influence the woman's posture.

First, there is the gradually increasing bulk and weight of pregnancy. In order to maintain balance during standing and walking, the mother must lean farther backward to counterbalance her altered weight distribution. The result of her postural adjustment is an increase in her lordosis. In the final weeks of pregnancy, the lordosis may become excessive, and this may lead to overstretching of the tissues surrounding the joints of the lower back (Fig. 8.1).

Second, to prepare the body for the impending delivery of the baby, the joints of the pelvis and lower back are made more flexible and elastic through a natural increase in certain hormones. The greater elasticity means that these joints become more lax and are easily overstretched when subjected to mechanical strains.

Once the child is born, the mother is often too busy to care for herself properly, and sometimes the postural fault that has developed during pregnancy remains for the rest of her life.

If your back problems began during or after pregnancy, it is possible that your lordosis has become excessive and that your problems are caused mostly by postural stresses. If this is the case, the extension exercises recommended for most people with lower back pain (Back Exercises 1 through 4) are unsuitable for you at the present time, and you should concentrate mainly on correcting your standing posture (Fig. 8.2). *Problems caused by postural stresses are always resolved by postural correction.*

For one week you must watch your posture very closely. At all times, maintain the correct posture, not only while standing but also while walking. You must *stand tall and walk tall* and not allow yourself to slouch. If, after one week of postural correction, the pain has disappeared or decreased considerably, faulty posture can be blamed for your back problems.

If your back problems began during or after pregnancy

Figure 8.1: Typical standing position in pregnancy

Figure 8.2: Correct standing posture

Figure 8.3: Flexion in Lying

Figure 8.4: Flexion in Sitting

and you *feel worse when standing and walking but much better when sitting*, extension exercises are not suitable for you. Now, in addition to the postural correction you maintain while standing and walking, perform the flexion exercises and self-treatment consisting of Back Exercises 5 and 6, Flexion in Lying (Fig. 8.3) and Flexion in Sitting (Fig. 8.4).

During the first week, perform Exercise 5 at regular intervals—that is, ten times per session and six to eight sessions per day. When you have improved to some extent with this procedure, add Exercise 6 in the second week. Exercise 6 must follow Exercise 5 and should be done with the same frequency. *Flexion exercises performed to relieve back pain appearing during pregnancy should not be followed by Back Exercise 3, Extension in Lying*. Once you are completely pain free, you may stop Exercise 5. In order to prevent recurrence of lower back problems, continue Exercise 6 twice per day, preferably in the morning and evening. At all times, maintain good postural habits, but do *not* use a lumbar roll.

If you are uncertain which category you belong in— someone who should use flexion exercises or someone who should use extension exercises—consult a credentialed member or associate of the McKenzie Institute.

CASE HISTORY: ADAPTATIONS FOR PREGNANCY

Martha is a thirty-three-year-old Georgia policewoman. She began to have lower back pain, radiating into the left thigh, five weeks into a pregnancy, and she knew of no reason for the symptoms. She had the pain while standing and sitting. She saw a doctor eighteen weeks into the pregnancy and was told, correctly, that she had a herniated nucleus pulposus.

She tried Back Exercise 4, Extension in Standing, but it had no effect. Her pregnancy did not permit her to do Exercise 3, Extension in Lying. But a McKenzie-credentialed physical therapist told her she could get most of the benefits of Exercise 3 by adapting it to her pregnancy. He had her stand about two feet from a wall and place her forearms against it. He then had her let her lower back sag as in Exercise 3. After she had done this just fifteen times in a single session, her symptoms stopped. Immediately after the exercise, the symptoms were still gone.

The pain would come back from time to time, but doing the adapted Exercise 3 at home helped. A lumbar roll made it possible for her to sit with better posture and less pain.

The same therapist adapted Back Exercise 5, Flexion in Lying, for use during Martha's pregnancy. Instead of having Martha pull both legs to her chest, the therapist instructed her to pull up one leg at a time. This caused her no pain, and the exercise helped in her recovery.

Throughout the remainder of her pregnancy she was able to keep her symptoms under control, primarily through use of the adapted version of Back Exercise 3.

LOWER BACK PAIN IN ATHLETES

After forty-five years of practice, I have come to the conclusion that lower back problems occurring in athletes—ranging from the professional to the recreational—require more than the usual amount of attention. The symptoms of lower back pain occurring in athletes can often behave in a fashion that is extremely mystifying and confusing. A combination of several factors adds to the confusion.

First, athletes are highly motivated to participate in their treatment and sometimes, in an attempt to speed their recovery, carry to excess the advice given to them. Their overexuberant participation in the rehabilitation of their back problems very often *delays rather than accelerates* the healing process.

A second important point is that the athlete's enthusiasm to participate in his or her favorite pastime or sport often leads him or her to return to full participation long before there has been sufficient time for complete healing.

A third and certainly the most common source of confusion can stem from the widespread belief among athletes that the sole cause of their problem lies in their frequent participation in a particular sporting activity. Later, this belief is reinforced by a health professional, who all too often comes to the same conclusion. It is not difficult to reach this conclusion, for probably three out of five athletes who experience lower back pain state that their pain appears after they have participated in a sport or have engaged in some equally vigorous activity.

All this comes from a mistaken effort at logic that plagues people who try to analyze their health care problems. The Latin for it is *post hoc, ergo propter hoc*, meaning "after this, therefore because of this." *Merriam-Webster's Collegiate Dictionary* defines the phrase as "relating to or being the fallacy of arguing from temporal sequence to a causal relation."

If your back began hurting an hour after your friend called you on the phone, would you say that the call with the friend injured your back? This is an extreme and silly example of the logical fallacy just described. But the fact is that people, including not just back sufferers but also their health care professionals, tend to believe that when back pain follows an activity that involves the back—even if it involves the back in good posture—the pain is due to the activity.

Many athletic careers have stopped for weeks or months or permanently because of *post hoc, ergo propter hoc*. Let's be sure that you don't stop your activity because of a logical fallacy. The belief that pain appearing shortly after activity must be caused by the activity itself is widespread and understandable but unfortunately it's frequently mistaken.

Often, the true cause of pain in athletes is that they adopt a slouched position after they have, in their athletic endeavor, thoroughly exercised their joints (Fig. 8.5). After exertion, we usually sit down and relax: because we are tired, we almost immediately adopt the relaxed sitting posture. In other words, after vigorously exercising, we collapse "in a heap" and slouch badly.

During vigorous exercise the joints of the spine are moved rapidly in many directions over an extended period of time. This process causes a thorough stretching in all directions of the soft tissues surrounding the joints. In addition, the fluid gel contained in the spinal discs is loosened, and it seems that distortion or displacement can occur if, after exercise, an exercised joint is placed in an extreme posture. This is very often the cause of back pain in athletes, and the cause-and-effect relationship can be proven rather easily, as will be explained.

If lower back pain has in fact occurred as a result of participation in a sport, it would be appropriate to recommend rest from the activity. But if the pain has appeared *after the activity has been completed and as a result of adopting a slouched sitting posture, resting would be entirely inappropriate.* To advise an athlete to cease participation in his or her favorite pastime can have serious consequences, both emotional and physical.

If you are an athlete, or if you participate in vigorous nonathletic activities, and you have recently developed lower back pain, it is necessary to discover the true cause of your problem. In order to treat your condition correctly and successfully, *we must determine whether your pain appeared during the particular activity or afterward.*

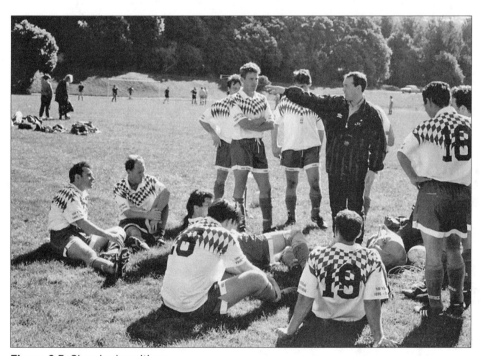

Figure 8.5: Slouched positions

If the pain appeared *during* the activity itself, your sport may well be the cause of the present problems. You may remember something that happened at the time of the activity and can describe what you felt at that moment. But

Figure 8.6: Lower back in moderate lordosis, supported by lumbar roll

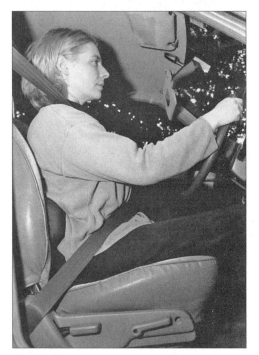

Figure 8.7: Driving with correct posture

a very large percentage of people who have back pain and participate in a sport never feel discomfort or pain while they are participating; their pain appears *after* the activity.

It's easy to determine if your lower back problems are the result of slouched sitting that occurred after an athletic or other activity. From now on, *immediately after the activity*, watch your posture closely and sit correctly with the lower back in a moderate lordosis and supported by a lumbar roll (Fig. 8.6).

For example, if you have finished a few sets of tennis, a game of football, or a round of golf, do not then sink into a comfortable lounge chair, slouch on a nearby patch of grass, or slouch in the car as you drive home. Instead, sit correctly, with your posture maintained precisely (Fig. 8.7). If, with this extra postural care, no pain occurs after a sports activity that previously was followed by back problems, the answer to your problem is clear and the responsibility for preventing further trouble is entirely your own.

If you fall into the group of people who develop pain only after activity, do not begin the McKenzie Method exercises at the same time that you begin correcting your posture. If the exercises are performed in conjunction with postural correction, it is impossible to determine whether you improved because of the postural correction or the exercises.

If your pain continues to appear after activity in spite of correcting your posture, it is possible that at some point during or before the activity you weakened or damaged some of the soft tissues in your lower back. If this is the case, *now* is the time to begin self-treatment. To do this, perform Back Exercises 3 and 4—Extension in Lying and Extension in Standing—on a regular basis.

Poor posture is often seen in athletes during intervals of nonparticipation: for example, when waiting their turn to come to the plate in baseball or to practice free throws in basketball. It is necessary to maintain good posture during these intervals as well as after completion of the activity.

If your pain appears regularly *while* you run or jog, you should begin the self-treatment program outlined in Chapter 7, "Instructions for People with Acute Lower Back Pain." You should also seek advice about the type of shoes you wear, the surfaces you run on, and, possibly, your running technique. If your problems persist despite following the advice in Chapter 7, you may need special treatment.

LOWER BACK PAIN IN THOSE OVER FIFTY

It is now known that acute lower back pain tends to occur less frequently in a person once we pass the age of fifty. So if you are over fifty (or even a little younger), you may notice that you experience a more persistent ache in the lower back than you previously had but that you no longer have the acute and severe episodes that affected you when you were younger. Nevertheless, this aching can cause significant problems, especially if it forces you to reduce activity. The human body thrives on activity and decays with prolonged inactivity. It is undesirable for any of us, regardless of age, to reduce our level of activity. Only if reduced activity is forced upon us by significant health-related problems should we exercise less.

CASE HISTORY: JOURNAL

Herb, a New York journalist, was also a long-distance runner. From age twenty-eight to thirty-four, he completed seven marathons; his only pain was from sore legs and a chafed toe. But during a vacation when he was forty-four, he ran one rigorous but short race (1.7 miles) in California's Sierra Nevada. He was pain free during the event, but was so exhausted by running hard at high altitude that, right after the race, he bent over for about two minutes, his hands on his knees. While doing this, he suddenly had severe pain in the middle of the lower back, pain that did not go away even when he resumed a normal standing posture.

Herb could not walk a step without sharp pain and needed a ride back to his car at the start of the race (he had planned to walk). He naturally assumed that running had caused the pain, and he was afraid he would have to give up this form of exercise. A cousin told Herb about the McKenzie Method and its explanation that when one has no pain while exercising but has pain directly thereafter, the culprit is almost always poor posture after exercise rather than the exercise itself: the exercise merely makes the athlete more vulnerable to the problems that can be caused by poor posture.

After doing his first set of McKenzie exercises, Herb's pain became much better; he was helped especially by Back Exercise 3, Extension in Lying, and Exercise 5, Flexion in Lying. He also learned the importance of maintaining good posture in standing or sitting after hard exercise. He soon was able to return to running. With attention to his postrunning posture, Herb never again had back pain following training runs or races.

A health professional may tell you that you have "degenerative" changes in your back or that you have arthritis and will "just have to live with it." *While it may be true that your back has become worn somewhat with aging, it certainly is not true that you will "just have to live with it."* It has been found that many people who have spinal joints that are worn with age have never had back pain, and we now know that the wear is not, by itself, a cause of pain.

In my experience, there are few people who would not derive some benefit from this book's advice about posture or the exercises, or both. Every older person should carry out the advice for correcting the sitting, standing, and lying postures.

Not all of you in the older group will be able to perform each exercise as advised, but all of you should *try*. I have found that age is not necessarily a barrier to the successful application of the exercises. Although there are some who may not succeed because of weakness or disability, most will be able to advance at least partway through the recommended program.

My advice to you is to consider starting the exercise program but with a reduced number of repetitions of the exercises you do in each session and to do fewer sessions in the course of a day. Don't hurry the process, and always rest adequately after completing the exercises—properly supported in the correct position, of course!

OSTEOPOROSIS

From middle age on, many women are affected by a disorder called osteoporosis. This is essentially a mineral-deficiency disorder. During menopause the body's calcium absorption rate drops significantly, and this deficiency continues throughout the years after menopause. Left untreated, calcium deficiency leads to a weakening of bone structure and a slow but progressive reduction in bone density. This in turn allows the posture of people with osteoporosis to become extremely rounded, especially in the middle—*thoracic*—part of the spine.

People affected by this disorder are at risk of suffering fractured vertebrae even without significant force being involved. Research conducted at the Mayo Clinic in the United States found that regularly performing extension exercises (Fig. 8.8) significantly reduced the number of compression fractures occurring in the group performing them. A similar group exercising differently and a group not exercising at all had significantly more fractures when examined at least one year after the beginning of the study. The Mayo study suggests that women from about the age of forty onward should practice extension exercises on a regular basis.

Here is how to do the exercise found so effective in the Mayo study:

Lie facedown with a pillow under your abdomen. With the hands clasped behind the neck or behind the lower back, lift the top half of your body. At the same time, lift both legs, remembering to keep them straight. After lifting the body and legs as high as possible, gradually lower both and relax for one second.

The exercise should be repeated until the back muscles feel fatigued and the exercise is becoming difficult to continue. The exercise should be performed fifteen to twenty times, four or five times per week, for about a month. After that time you should gradually increase the number of exercises until you are doing fifty to sixty at a time. You should do the Mayo exercise for the rest of your life!

If you are uncertain how to follow this advice, discuss it with your doctor before beginning the program. If you have difficulties with the exercises for one reason or another, consult a McKenzie-credentialed physical therapist or chiropractor who can show you ways to modify the exercises without necessarily reducing their effectiveness.

The muscles you strengthen by doing the exercise recommended by the Mayo Clinic study are also the muscles responsible for holding you upright. Maintaining good posture at all times will probably assist in the strengthening process. Good posture may also reduce the likelihood of small fractures occurring.

Figure 8.8: Mayo Clinic exercise

9 COMMON BACK REMEDIES AND SOLUTIONS

MEDICINES AND DRUGS

As mentioned earlier in this book, most of the common back pains we experience are mechanical in origin and therefore are affected only by those drugs and medications that are able to relieve pain. There are no medicines or drugs able to remove the *causes* of our common backaches and pains. Therefore, medication should be taken only when your pains are severe or when you must find relief.

Certain medications, such as aspirin and other nonsteroidal anti-inflammatory drugs (NSAIDs), have been found to be the most useful for alleviating acute back pain and have fewer side effects than some commonly prescribed medications. Both have been recommended by the U.S. government's Agency for Health Care Policy and Research (now the Agency for Healthcare Research and Quality).

BED REST

When your back pain is so severe that bed rest is required, you should restrict this period of rest, if at all possible, to two or three days.

A study conducted in the United States demonstrated that patients who rested in bed for two days recovered as well as those who stayed in bed for seven days. But patients who continued to walk and move were able to go back to work sooner than those who rested for either two or seven days. (R. A. Deyo et al., 1986, "How Many Days of Bed Rest for Acute Low Back Pain?" *New England Journal of Medicine* 315:1064–70.) And I have seen many patients who could still not get out of bed after ten days.

ACUPUNCTURE

Acupuncture can relieve pain and, when all else has failed, is well worth a try. You should be aware, however, that as with taking medications, acupuncture can give you relief, but it cannot correct the underlying mechanical problem.

BACK PAIN IN THE COMMUNITY

Lower back pain is widespread throughout the world, both in Western and Eastern cultures. In Western countries, in which more data are available, approximately 80 percent of people will at least one time in their lives suffer a back pain episode so severe as to require bed rest.

Many things could be done to improve this situation. You as an individual should complain whenever you find inappropriate seating in public offices or buildings or in public transit vehicles. If your car's seats are inadequate, you should complain to your car dealer; better still, look for another car or consider having your car retrofitted with better seats.

I was about to write, "When choosing lounge furniture . . . ," but an American friend of mine has advised me that in the United States a "lounge" is generally a bar or a women's rest room. So I will rephrase. I mean to comment on furniture used for relaxing at home. So I will say that when choosing *living room* furniture (which nearly always seems designed to cause or perpetuate back problems), you should persist until you find chairs that are properly designed. When you are in a furniture store and find seating that is poorly designed, you should tell the manager that this is the case. If you complain to a car dealer or a furniture store manager, nothing will change instantly. But enough complaints can result in reform.

Few airlines provide seating that adequately supports the lower back. This has serious consequences for some individuals who must fly long distances and for many hours.

Office workers should demand seating that provides adequate lumbar support. There are many sophisticated-looking and expensive office and secretarial chairs on the market that provide no lumbar support whatsoever. On the other hand, chairs that provide good support can often be found at moderate prices.

Although poor seating design is a major factor contributing to the development of lower back pain, another, more important factor is becoming increasingly evident. Where once our school physical education instructors were concerned with poor posture in our children and corrected it when they saw it, they now seem more interested in producing the best football team, the highest-scoring basketball player, and the fastest sprinter. Physical education teachers in all parts of the world no longer seem to equip our children with the information that is so necessary if they are to care for their own physical needs during a lifetime on this planet.

Spinal pain of postural origin would not occur if this basic education were given to individuals at an early age. Ask any twelve-year-old child if he or she has been shown at school how to stand correctly or how to sit correctly. Chances are that the child will tell you that he or she has never been shown either of these two fundamental postures. Similarly, chances are slim that the child has been told about the harmful consequences that may occur if posture is neglected.

If these matters are of concern to you, you might politely request that your school administration or P.E. teachers make postural physical education a priority. In addition, you might suggest that administrators evaluate school furniture for its effects on posture. Good postural habits must be instilled at an early age.

These are steps that you as a concerned individual can take to help bring about some of the changes that must occur if society is to grapple sensibly with the enormous problem of back pain. In the United States alone, this problem costs $50 to $70 billion a year in everything from medical expenses to days lost from work.

For information on the McKenzie Institute's posture correction video, which is available to schools, please see Appendix A.

10 NECK PROBLEMS

NECK PROBLEMS COME WITH MANY NAMES. ARTHRITIS IN THE NECK. Spondylosis of the neck. Rheumatism. Fibrositis. Slipped disc. And, when they involve pain extending into the arm, neuritis and neuralgia.

At some time during our lives, most of us suffer from pain in the neck or from pain originating in the neck that is felt across the shoulders, in a shoulder blade, or in the upper or lower arm. Pain coming from the neck can also be felt as far away as the hand, and symptoms such as "pins and needles" and numbness can be felt in the fingers. Some people suffer from headaches that can be traced to problems in the neck.

Usually the aches and pains occur intermittently. That is, there are times in the day when no pain is felt, or there are whole days when no pain is felt. The symptoms may appear mysteriously, often for no apparent reason. And just as enigmatically the symptoms may vanish.

These aches and pains also may occur constantly. That is, some patients experience pain at all times, to one degree or another. Often people in this situation find they have to resort to taking pain pills. Although it is uncommon for these people to have to stop work, even this occasionally does occur. More often, the pain simply makes their lives miserable and they must reduce their activities in order to keep their discomfort at a moderate level. Therefore neck problems can seriously affect their lifestyle.

If you have neck problems, you may already have discovered that symptoms can in some cases last for months or even years. Or you may have found treatments that stop your pain, but the pain returns later. You may be reading this book because you have persistent pain that has not disappeared, despite the fact that you have received the best of treatment.

Whatever the situation, you have most likely realized that many of the treatments that doctors, physical therapists, and chiropractors prescribe address only your present symptoms and are not directed at preventing future problems. Time and again you may have to seek assistance to get relief from your neck pain.

How good it would be if you were able to treat yourself whenever the pain returned! Better yet, how good it would be if you could apply a system of treatment to yourself that would prevent the pain from coming back!

But I am not writing about some dream world that does not exist; I am not describing some old black-and-white episode of *The Twilight Zone*. In fact, since around the early 1970s, many effective methods have been developed that enable us to manage our own spinal problems. Unfortunately, this information has been treated like a well-kept secret. It was not widely disseminated among health professionals until the 1980s. This is because, like many developments in medicine, new ideas must be shown to be effective before they are widely adopted.

The method I have developed has been used by doctors and physical therapists in many parts of the world since the early 1970s, and generally their patients are achieving the same happy results.

One of the main points of this book is that, just as with the back, the management of the neck is *your* responsibility. If, for some reason or other, *you* have developed neck problems, then *you* must learn how to deal with your present symptoms and how to prevent future problems. Self-treatment will be more effective in the long-term management of your neck pain than any other form of therapy.

Despite its value to most neck patients, this book is not meant for you, at least not at this stage, if you have developed neck pain for the first time and it is no better ten days after onset. In that case, consult your doctor, who will evaluate your neck problems from various medical angles. When appropriate, he or she will refer you to a physical therapist (ideally a McKenzie-credentialed one) for treatment and, more important, for advice and instructions on how to prevent further neck problems. You should also seek advice from your doctor if there are complications to your neck problems. Examples of complications are severe, stabbing pains; your head being pulled off center; or severe, continuing headaches.

Finally, this book will help 80 percent of people with neck pain, which is to say that it will not help 20 percent. This book is meant for those with straightforward mechanical problems, which are by far the most common cause of neck pain. I hope you fall into this category and that you will therefore benefit greatly from this book.

THE CERVICAL SPINE

The technical name for the series of vertebrae in the neck is the *cervical spine*. As you will recall from Chapter 2, the spine (Fig. 10.1) consists of thirty-three bones called vertebrae. The top seven are the cervical vertebrae. These rest upon one another like a stack of spools. Each vertebra has a solid part in front, called the vertebral body, and a hole in the back (Fig. 10.2). When lined up as the spinal column, these holes form the spinal canal. This canal serves as a protected passageway for the spinal cord, the bundle of nerves that extends from head to pelvis.

Separating the vertebrae are special cartilage structures called discs. These are located between the vertebral bodies, just in front of the spinal cord (Fig. 10.3). Each disc consists of a soft fluid center part, the *nucleus*. The nucleus is surrounded and held together by a cartilage ring, called the *annulus* or *annular ligament*. The discs are like rubber washers and act as shock absorbers. They are able to alter their shape, thus allowing movement of one vertebra on another and allowing movement of the neck as a whole.

The vertebrae and the discs are linked by a series of joints to form the cervical spine. Each joint is held together by its surrounding soft tissues, that is, by a capsule reinforced by ligaments. Muscles lie over one or more joints of the neck and may extend upward to the head or downward to the trunk. At each end, each muscle changes into a tendon by which it attaches itself to different bones. When a muscle contracts, it causes movement in one or more joints.

Between each two vertebrae are two small openings, one on either side. Through these openings, the left and right spinal nerves leave the spinal canal (Fig. 10.3). Among other tasks, the spinal nerves supply our muscles with power and our skin with sensation. The nerves are really part of our alarm system: pain is the warning that a structure is about to be damaged or has already sustained some damage.

Figure 10.1: The human spine viewed from the side

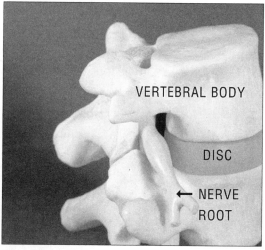

Figure 10.2: A vertebra

Figure 10.3: Two vertebrae

FUNCTIONS OF THE CERVICAL SPINE

On top of this complex of bones and "washers" rests the head. The head contains our computer system, better known as the brain, as well as important sensors associated with it, such as the eyes, ears, nose, and mouth. The vertebrae, the discs, and the head form a series of flexible joints that allow the head to turn almost 180 degrees from one side to the other, to look up and down, and to tilt left and right. In addition, the head can adopt many positions that are combinations of the movements mentioned above.

The main functions of the cervical spine are:

- To support the head
- To allow it to move in many directions and adjust its position in fine degrees in order to assist the working of the sensors
- To provide a protected passageway for the bundle of nerves that extends from the brain to the sacrum, which is the tail end of the spine

The neck has a high degree of flexibility due to the "specially designed" structure of the joints, in particular those between the uppermost vertebrae and the head. Its flexibility is further increased because in this area no bony structures are attached to the spine. Therefore the neck can move relatively more freely than the rest of the spine, whose movements are restricted by the rib cage and the pelvis. On the other hand, because the neck is not surrounded and supported by these structures, it is also more vulnerable than the rest of the spine when it is subjected to strains. The very flexibility of the neck, so helpful and so necessary for everyday living, is also the cause of many of our problems. The wide range of movement of the neck exposes it to an equally wide range of stresses and strains.

NATURAL POSTURE

A side view of the human body shows that there is a small inward curve in the neck just above the shoulder girdle. Can you guess what this inward curve is called? It's a word you certainly have heard enough in this book. Yes, it's called a lordosis. When we discussed the back, we repeatedly referred to the *lumbar* lordosis. The inward curve in your neck is called the *cervical* lordosis. This curve in the cervical spine is our main concern in this "neck part" of this book.

The shoulder girdle consists of the left and right *scapulae* (shoulder blades) and the left and right *clavicles* (collarbones). When you stand upright, your head should be directly above the shoulder girdle, thereby forming a small but visible lordosis (Fig. 10.4). Due to postural neglect, people can often be seen with the head in front of the body, with the chin poking forward (Fig. 10.5). When this is the case, the cervical lordosis is altered in shape and the joints are distorted. In this position, the joints of the lower neck are bent relatively forward (flexed), whereas the joints between the upper part of the neck and the head are bent backward (extended). This is called the "protruded head posture" and, if present often enough and for long enough, it can cause neck pain to develop.

WHY NECK PAIN?

Mechanical pain occurs when the joint between two bones has been placed in a position that overstretches the surrounding soft tissues. This is true for

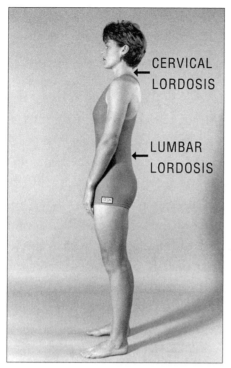

CERVICAL LORDOSIS

LUMBAR LORDOSIS

Figure 10.4: Good posture, featuring the cervical lordosis

Figure 10.5: Bad posture, with the head protruding

mechanical pain in any joint of the body, but in the spine there are additional factors. Here the tissues that surround the joints between the vertebrae, in particular the tissues in the ligaments, are also responsible for supporting the soft discs that separate the vertebrae. These tissues hold the discs in an enclosed compartment and help to form a shock-absorbing mechanism.

Pain of mechanical origin may arise in the neck for the following reasons:

- The ligaments and other soft tissues that hold the vertebrae together may simply be overstretched but without further damage.
- An outside force may cause overstretching by placing a sudden, severe strain on the neck. Examples are injuries sustained in auto accidents and contact sports. This type of stress cannot always be avoided, as it occurs unexpectedly and takes a person unawares.
- Most often, postural stresses that place less severe strains on the neck over a longer period of time cause the overstretching. This type of stress

is one that *we exert on our own neck*, and therefore we can easily influence it. Here lies our main responsibility in the self-treatment and prevention of neck pain.

Complications arise when overstretching of soft tissues leads to actual tissue damage. It is often thought that neck pain is caused by strained muscles. Muscles, which are the source of power and movement, can indeed be overstretched and thereby injured. But muscle injury requires a considerable amount of external force and does not happen all that often. In addition, muscles usually heal rapidly and seldom cause pain lasting for more than a week or two.

On the other hand, whenever the impact of the injuring force is severe enough to affect the muscles, the underlying soft tissues, such as the capsule and ligaments, will be damaged as well. In fact, usually these two are damaged long before the muscles are. When these tissues heal, they may form scar tissue, become less elastic, and shorten. At this stage even normal movements may stretch the scars in these shortened structures and produce pain. Unless appropriate exercises are performed to gradually stretch and lengthen these structures and restore their normal flexibility, they may become a continuous source of neck pain or headache.

Complications of another nature arise when the ligaments surrounding a disc are injured to such an extent that the disc loses its ability to absorb shock and its outer wall is weakened. This allows the soft inside of the disc to bulge outward and, in extreme cases, to burst through the outer ligament, which may cause serious problems. When the disc bulge protrudes far enough backward, it may press painfully on the spinal nerve. This may cause some of the pains felt well away from the source of the trouble, for example in the arm or hand.

Due to this bulging, the disc may become severely distorted and prevent the vertebrae from lining up properly during movement. In this case, some movements may be blocked partially or completely, and forcing these movements causes severe pain. This is the reason that some people can hold the head only in an off-center position. Those of you who experience a sudden onset of pain and, following this, are unable to move the head in a normal way may have some bulging of the soft disc material. This need not be cause for alarm. The movements described in this book, and especially the seven exercises for the neck, are carefully designed to reduce any disturbance of this nature.

POSTURAL STRESSES

The most common form of neck pain is caused by the overstretching of ligaments due to postural stresses. This may occur when you sit with poor posture for a long time (Fig. 10.6); when you lie or sleep through the night with your head in an awkward position (Figs. 10.7a and 10.7b), and when you work in a strained position (Fig. 10.8).

Of all these postural stresses, the one that is by far most often at fault is poor sitting posture, that is, sitting with the head protruded. Poor posture may produce neck pain all by itself. But once neck problems have developed, poor posture will frequently make them worse and will always make them last longer than they otherwise would have.

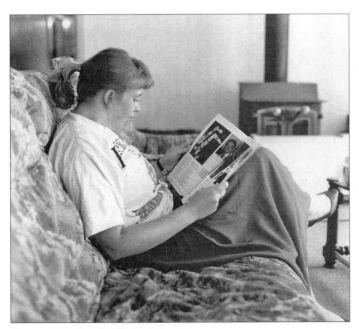

Figure 10.6: Bad sitting posture

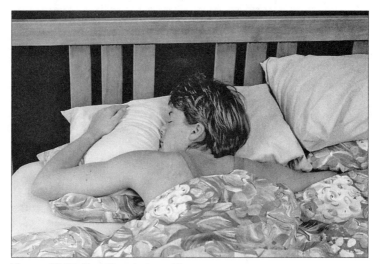

Figure 10.7a: Bad sleeping position

Figure 10.7b: Bad lying position

The main theme of this chapter is that if you avoid prolonged overstretching, pain of postural origin will not occur. If pain does develop, there are certain movements—and in particular certain exercises—you can perform in order to stop the pain. You should not have to seek assistance whenever postural pain arises.

Figure 10.8: Strained working position

WHERE THE PAIN IS FELT

The sites of pain caused by neck problems vary from one person to another. In a first attack, pain is usually felt at or near the base of the neck, in the center (Fig. 10.9) or just to one side (Fig. 10.10). Usually the pain subsides within a few days. In subsequent attacks, pain may reach across both shoulders (Fig. 10.11), to the top of one shoulder, or to the shoulder blade (Fig. 10.12). Later still, pain may reach the outside or back of the upper arms as far as the elbow (Fig. 10.13), or it may extend below the elbow to the wrist or hand, and you may feel "pins and needles" or numbness in the fingers (Fig. 10.14). As a result of neck problems, some people experience headaches. Often these headaches are felt at the top of the neck and at the base and back of the head, on one or both sides (Fig. 10.15). But they also can spread from the back of the head over the top of the head to above or behind the eye, again on one or both sides (Fig. 10.16).

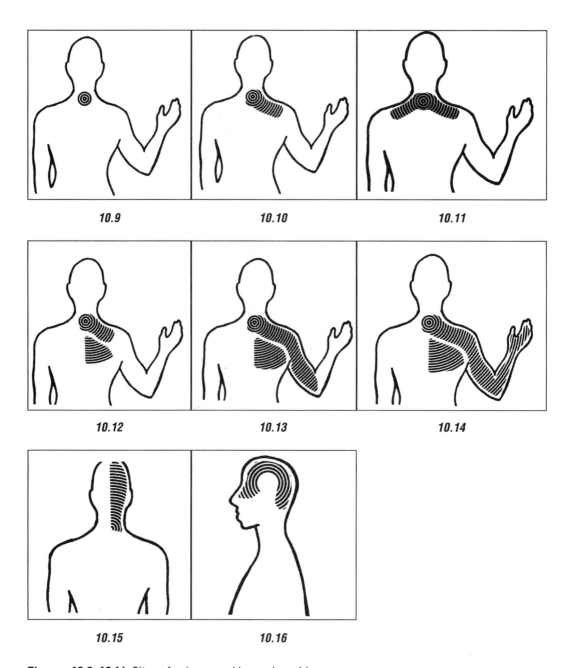

Figures 10.9–10.16: Sites of pain caused by neck problems

WHO CAN PERFORM SELF-TREATMENT?

Only relatively few people with neck pain will not benefit from the advice given in this book. Nearly everyone can begin the exercise program, provided the recommended precautions are taken. Once you have started the exercises, carefully watch your pain pattern. If your pain is getting progressively worse, and it remains worse the following day, you should stop the exercises and get advice from your doctor or McKenzie-credentialed physical therapist. In any of the following situations, *do not begin the exercise program* without first consulting your doctor or physical therapist:

- If you have developed neck pain for the first time and it is no better ten days after onset.
- If you have pain near or at the wrist or hand and experience sensations of "pins and needles" or numbness in the fingers.
- If you have developed neck problems following a recent, severe accident.
- If you have recently developed headaches. In this case, your eyes or eyeglasses may need to be checked.
- If you experience severe headaches that have come on for no apparent reason, have never gone away, and are gradually getting worse.
- If you have episodes of severe headaches that are accompanied by nausea and dizziness.

11 COMMON CAUSES OF NECK PAIN

SITTING FOR PROLONGED PERIODS

When we are moving about, especially when we walk briskly, we assume a fairly upright posture. Our head is retracted and held directly over the vertebral column and consequently receives the maximum possible support. When we sit and relax in a chair (Fig. 11.1a), the head and neck slowly protrude, because the muscles that support them get tired. As the muscles tire, they relax, and we lose the main support for good posture.

The result is the protruded head posture (Fig. 11.1b). We see this posture around us every day. It is not present during infancy but develops from the midteen years onward. We are not really designed to sit for six to eight hours daily, five to six days a week.

When the protruded head posture is maintained long enough, it causes overstretching of the ligaments. As a result, pain will arise *only in certain positions.* Once the protruded posture has become a habit and is maintained most of the time, it may also cause distortion of the discs in the vertebral joints. At this stage, *movements as well as positions* will produce pain. Neck problems developed this way are the result of postural neglect. Poor neck

Figure 11.1a: Bad sitting posture   **Figure 11.1b:** Protruded head posture

posture is not the only cause of neck pain. It is, however, one of the main causes and it is the most troublesome factor in causing neck pain to go on and on.

When you sit, the position of the lower back strongly influences the posture of the neck. If the lower back is allowed to slouch, it is impossible to sit with the head and neck pulled backward. You can easily verify this for yourself. Unfortunately, once we have been sitting in a certain position for a few minutes, our body sags and we end up sitting slouched with a rounded lower back *and* a protruded head and neck. For most people, sitting for long periods results in sitting with poor posture.

Environmental Factors

The design of seating found in business and industrial settings, transportation, and the home only encourages poor postural habits. Rarely do the chairs and seats available give adequate support to the lower back and neck; instead, unless we make a conscious effort to sit correctly, they allow us (or even force us) to sit badly.

CASE HISTORY: BEHIND THE EIGHT BALL

Rikki is a thirty-eight-year-old factory worker in Michigan. For three months before beginning the McKenzie program, she had pain in the neck, left shoulder, and upper left arm. She said her neck pain was an 8 on a scale of 0 to 10.

The pain would get worse during the day. In her job, she sat on a stool with no back. She had to lean over a bench and install small wires in electric motors. She had extremely poor posture, and her McKenzie-credentialed physical therapist performed a manual correction of the lumbar spine while Rikki was sitting. This immediately improved Rikki's posture and reduced her neck pain; the patient now said the level of pain was a 4.

The physical therapist introduced Rikki to the McKenzie exercises, in particular the slouch-overcorrect movements for posture and Neck Exercise 1, Head Retraction in Sitting. This exercise allowed Rikki to almost eliminate her arm and shoulder pain. Her neck pain centralized and declined to what she rated as a 3. At home, she continued with the slouch-overcorrect procedure and Neck Exercise 1.

In her second physical therapy visit, Rikki progressed to Neck Exercise 2, Neck Extension in Sitting. With her hands, she added "overpressure" to the exercise (see Chapter 12), resulting in greater extension. As a result of Neck Exercises 1 and 2, her symptoms were completely resolved. After six visits with the McKenzie therapist, Rikki was able to complete an eight-hour workday without any symptoms recurring. She remained on a home program of postural correction and neck exercise. As a result, she remained pain free.

For the neck, ideally the back of your chair comes up high enough that you can rest your head against it. But many seats provide no support for the head. An exception are the seats manufactured for most airlines, but, unfortunately, their head support pushes the head and neck into the very same protruded position that causes our problems. It is the brave person indeed who takes the risk of sleeping in one of these seats, because when this person wakes up he or she may well feel the old familiar pains in the neck.

When traveling by car, train, bus, or plane, we often are compelled to sit in the position dictated by the seats provided. It may be necessary for the driver of a car, bus, or truck to protrude the head and neck in order to see through the windshield; this is especially likely in bad weather.

Furniture in offices and factories all over the world is often designed poorly. Improvements have been made in the past decade, but not enough. And, to make matters worse, the furniture is rarely adaptable to individual requirements. This is one of the reasons that so many people who spend most of their day in a seated working position develop lower back and neck pain. Until all furniture designers understand the requirements of the human frame and begin to manufacture their chairs accordingly, we will continue to suffer from their neglect.

Finally, the design of domestic furniture is not any better. Unless your favorite living room chair is exceptional, you will have insufficient support in the lower back and the neck and will continue to place strains on these areas when you relax in the evening. If your neck problems are aggravated by reading or watching television, it is unlikely that the story is what's giving you a pain in the neck. The cause of the pain is not a ridiculous plot or unconvincing acting but rather the posture you have adopted. And this posture depends to a large extent on the type of chair or support you use.

Although the poor design of furniture contributes to the development of back problems, equal blame lies with the way we use the furniture. If we do not know how to sit correctly, even the best-designed chairs will not prevent us from slouching. On the other hand, once we are reeducated in correct sitting, bad chairs will not have a big impact on our posture.

How to Manage Prolonged Sitting Situations

In order to *prevent the development of neck pain* due to sitting poorly for long periods, you will need to (1) sit correctly and (2) interrupt at regular intervals the protruded head posture or prolonged bending of the neck.

In order to *treat neck pain* resulting from poor posture, you may need to perform other exercises in addition to correcting your posture. In this chapter I will discuss only the exercises required to reduce postural stresses and to correct your posture. The exercises for relief of pain and for increase of function will be described in the next chapter.

Correcting the Sitting Posture

You may have been sitting slouched for many years without neck and shoulder pain. But once you have developed neck problems, you must no longer sit in the old way, because the slouched posture will only continue the overstretching discussed previously.

If you are sitting slouched, with the lower back rounded, it is not possible to correct the posture of the neck (Fig. 11.2). Therefore you must *first correct the posture of your lower back.* Ideally, you will now review Chapter 4, "Common Causes of Lower Back Pain," and especially its advice on how to improve your posture when you sit and stand.

For the purposes of this chapter, however, you must be fully aware of the following. The lumbar lordosis, the natural hollow present in your lower back when you stand, must be maintained during sitting in order for you to sit correctly (Fig. 11.3). To achieve this, *the use of a lumbar roll is essential.* A lumbar roll is a specially designed support for your lower back (Fig. 11.4). The roll should be no more than four to five inches (about ten to thirteen centimeters) in diameter before being compressed, and it should be filled with foam of

Figure 11.2: Bad neck posture resulting from insufficient lower back support

Figure 11.3: Good neck posture made possible by use of a lumbar roll

moderate density. Without this support, your lower back slouches and your head protrudes as soon as you relax or concentrate on anything other than your posture. Examples are when you talk, read, write, watch TV, and drive your car. To counteract this slouching, you must place the lumbar roll in the small of your back at the level of your beltline; you must do this whenever you sit in an easy chair (Fig. 11.5), car (Fig. 11.6), or office chair (Figs. 11.7a and 11.7b).

Figure 11.4: Lumbar roll

You may purchase a lumbar roll made specifically for the above purpose from the authorized firm listed in Appendix B of this book. You will need to supply your waist measurement and your weight.

In order to correct your neck's posture when you sit, you must first learn *how to retract your head.* Therefore you must become fully practiced in Neck Exercise 1, Head Retraction in Sitting (see Chapter 12). You should perform this exercise fifteen to twenty times per session, and you should perform the session three times per day, preferably morning, noon, and evening. The

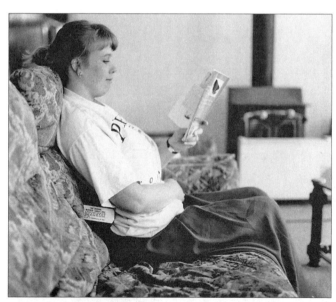

Figure 11.5: A lumbar roll enables you to counteract slouching when you sit in an easy chair.

Figure 11.6: Use of lumbar roll to correct poor car seat design

Figure 11.7a: Poor office chair design uncorrected

Figure 11.7b: Poor office chair design corrected by lumbar roll

rhythmic procedure of the exercise (remember to slowly say "pressure on, pressure off"; see Chapter 4) teaches you the correct position of your head in relation to your body.

Each backward movement of the head must be performed to the maximum possible degree. When you have pulled your head back as far as possible, you have assumed the retracted head posture (Fig. 11.8). Now you have reached the extreme of the corrected head and neck posture.

Once you know how to retract your head, you must learn *how to find and maintain the correct head and neck posture.* The extreme of the retracted head position is a position of strain and it is not possible to sit this way for long. To sit comfortably and correctly, you must hold your head just short of the extreme retracted posture. To find this position, first retract the head as far as possible (Fig. 11.8), then release the last 10 percent of this movement (Fig. 11.9). Now you have reached the correct head and neck posture, which can be maintained for any length of time. It may take up to a week or so of practice to master this. The aim of this part of the program is to first restore

Figure 11.8: "Retracted head posture"

Figure 11.9: After retracting the head, release the last 10 percent of movement.

the correct posture and then to maintain it. As a rule, the pain will decrease as your head posture improves, and you will have no pain once you maintain the correct posture. The pain will readily recur in the first few weeks whenever you allow your head to protrude. But eventually you will remain completely pain free, even when you accidentally forget your posture.

Even so, you should never again allow yourself to sit for long periods in a slouched position with your head protruded. As soon as you have been completely pain free for a couple of days, you can resume your normal activities. If from now on you follow the instructions in this book, you may also be able to prevent further neck trouble.

When you first use the above procedures to correct your lower back and neck posture in sitting, you will experience some new pains. These may differ from your original pain and may be felt in a new location. New pains are the result of performing new exercises and maintaining new positions. They should be expected and will wear off in a few days, provided postural correction is continued on a regular basis. Once you have become used to sitting correctly, you will enjoy it. You soon will notice the reduction or absence of pain and will experience an increased level of comfort. From then on, you will automatically choose chairs that allow you to sit correctly.

> **RULE:** When sitting for long periods, you must sit correctly, with the lower back supported by a lumbar roll and the head retracted.

Regularly Interrupting Prolonged Bending of the Neck

If you spend long periods of time in the sitting position—for example, while working at a desk or knitting—it is likely that, even with the best intentions, you will eventually forget to maintain the correct posture. Gradually you will assume a more or less protruded head posture or a position in which both head and neck are bent forward. To counteract this, you must frequently interrupt the forward-bent position by correcting your neck posture and stretching your head and neck backward (see Neck Exercise 2 in Chapter 12). This will relieve the stresses on the discs between the vertebrae as well as on the surrounding tissues.

> **RULE:** When sitting for long periods, it is essential to regularly interrupt prolonged bending of the neck. You can achieve this by retracting the head and extending the neck five or six times at regular intervals, for example, once an hour.

LYING DOWN AND RESTING

Other than sitting, the most frequent cause of neck pain is postural stress in the lying position. If you wake up in the morning with a stiff and painful neck that was not causing problems the night before, there is likely to be something wrong with the surface on which you are lying or with the position in which you are sleeping. It's a comparatively easy task to correct the surface on which you are lying but rather difficult to influence the position you adopt while sleeping. Once you are asleep, you may just regularly change your position or you may toss and turn. Unless a certain position causes so much discomfort that it wakes you up, you have no real idea of the various positions you assume while sleeping.

CASE HISTORY: WHAT A HEADACHE

Colleen, from Ohio, is a twenty-seven-year-old customer service agent with an airline. She had pain in the neck and the right shoulder blade. There was no known cause for the pain. The pain radiated down her right arm to her thumb and she had occasional headaches. When she started the McKenzie program, she had had these symptoms for about two months and they had gotten worse for three weeks. Activities that were painful included looking down, writing, being a passenger in a car, and turning her head, especially to the left. Her sleep was disturbed.

Colleen's neck's range of motion was limited. With McKenzie postural techniques, including use of a lumbar roll, her sitting posture improved and her neck and shoulder blade pain declined. Neck Exercise 1, Head Retraction in Sitting, reduced her symptoms and they remained better. She used a cervical roll for sleeping.

Four days after beginning the McKenzie program, Colleen had less neck pain and her headaches were less frequent and less intense. The cervical roll had enabled her to sleep without pain. Her range of motion had improved.

Three days later, the headaches were gone. Colleen noticed shoulder blade pain only when she woke up. She still had some pain when returning to a normal head position after looking down.

She began using the slouch-overcorrect technique to further improve her posture. Two weeks later Colleen was free of pain and had full range of motion.

Correcting the Surface for Lying Down

All that is required to correct the surface on which you are lying is to use a different pillow. You may need to change the material, the thickness, or both. You must realize that the main function of the pillow is to *support both head and neck.* Therefore it should fill the natural hollow in the contour of the neck between the head and shoulder girdle without tilting the head or lifting it up. The head itself should be allowed to rest in a dish-shaped hollow.

It follows that you must easily be able to adjust the contents of the pillow. Ideally your pillow will be made of feathers or down.

By pulling and pushing the contents of the pillow, you can make a hollow for your neck and bunch the edge to form a thick support for your neck. Pillows made of molded rubber or foam plastic, including specially designed cervical pillows made of memory foam, cannot be adjusted; their contents are fixed. They always adopt the shape of their original mold, regardless of attempts to change them, and this may not be suitable for your particular weight or shape. They do not permit the head to rest in a dish-shaped hollow but tend to apply a recoil pressure against the natural position the head would like to adopt. If you have such a pillow, you should replace it.

Figure 11.10: Soft foam cervical roll . . .

Figure 11.11a: . . . positioned inside a pillowcase . . .

If your pillow is made of a recommended material but still does not provide adequate support for your neck, you should also use a supportive roll. A roll used for the neck is called a cervical roll. Make a soft foam roll of about three inches (about eight centimeters) in diameter and eighteen inches (about forty-five centimeters) long (Fig. 11.10). Place this inside your pillowcase, on top of the pillow and along its lower border (Fig. 11.11a).

Alternatively, you can use a small hand towel of about twenty inches (about fifty centimeters) long and wide. Fold the towel in half and roll it loosely, then wind it around your neck and pin the ends together at the front. In both cases, the supportive roll will fill the space between the pillow and the neck (Fig. 11.11b). The measurements given above are merely a guide. All neck supports must fulfill individual requirements, and each person needs to experiment for himself or herself.

You may purchase the Original McKenzie cervical roll made specifically for the above purpose from the authorized firm listed in Appendix B of this book. You will need to provide your neck measurement and your weight. Place the roll inside your pillowcase, on top of the pillow, and along its lower edge.

Figure 11.11b: . . . in order to support the neck.

Correcting the Lying Posture

If the lying posture itself is thought to cause neck pain, it needs to be investigated for each person individually, largely by trial and error. Consult a credentialed member or associate of the McKenzie Institute (see Appendix A). But there is one position that requires further discussion. Some people like to sleep lying facedown; many of these people frequently wake up with a pain in the neck or with a headache, but the pain wears off as the day progresses. Other than this, they seem to have no neck problems.

When a person is lying facedown, the head is usually turned to one side. In this position some of the joints, especially in the upper neck, reach the maximum possible degree of turning or come very close to it (Fig. 11.12). Consequently, this position places great strain on the soft tissues surrounding the joints of the neck and the soft tissues of the joints between the upper neck and the head.

If you sleep lying facedown and awake with pain in the neck or with a headache, you must avoid lying facedown. In addition, you

Figure 11.12: This sleeping position causes excessive strain.

should perform exercises for the neck, in particular Neck Exercises 1, 2, and 6 (see Chapter 12). This is to ensure that you can retract the head and extend the neck properly and that you have an adequate range of movement when turning the head.

RELAXING AFTER VIGOROUS ACTIVITY

When you have finished a vigorous activity—for example, playing football or tennis or chopping wood—and have not suffered any pain as a result, *you should not relax by sitting or lying with the head in a protruded posture* (Figs. 11.13 and 11.14). Thoroughly exercised spinal joints easily distort if they are held in an overstretched position for a long period. A commonly heard story is that when a person sits down to rest following demanding exercise or hard work, sometime later the person has such severe pain that he or she can hardly move the neck. As with people who suffer back pain not long after playing a sport, usually people blame the exercise or work for their neck pain, but usually the pain has actually been produced by prolonged forward bending of the head and neck.

Figures 11.13–11.14: After a vigorous activity, do not relax by sitting or lying with the head in a protruded position.

WORKING IN AWKWARD POSITIONS OR CRAMPED SPACES

Some jobs can be performed only in positions that are likely to cause over-stretching of the neck. These jobs may require you to sit, and usually they involve precision work. Alternatively, they may have to be performed in cramped spaces or with the head and neck in an awkward static (unmoving) position. Under these circumstances, you may not be able to prevent the onset of neck pain just by regularly assuming the correct posture. If your neck problems are brought on by a job of the nature just described, you must, in addition to correcting your posture, frequently interrupt your overstretching and perform Neck Exercise 6, followed by Neck Exercises 1 and 2 (see Chapter 12).

RULE: When working with head and neck in a static position, interrupt this position at regular intervals by assuming the correct posture. In addition, perform five or six movements of Neck Exercise 6, then Neck Exercises 1 and 2 (see Chapter 12).

OSTEOPOROSIS

Beginning in middle age, many women are affected by osteoporosis. This is essentially a mineral-deficiency disorder. Although it affects the back more commonly than the neck, osteoporosis can cause symptoms in the neck as well.

For a more complete discussion of osteoporosis, see Chapter 8, "Special Back Situations." In particular, see that chapter's discussion of the Mayo Clinic study that showed that extension exercises reduced the incidence of compression fractures in the back. One can infer from the Mayo study that people suffering from osteoporosis of the neck would reduce their incidence of pain and injury if they were to do the neck extension exercises described in this book. All the neck exercises in this book except Neck Exercise 7 are extension exercises.

12 THE MCKENZIE METHOD EXERCISES FOR THE NECK

GENERAL GUIDELINES AND PRECAUTIONS

The McKenzie neck exercise program consists of seven exercises. The McKenzie *back* exercise program consists of seven different exercises; you will find them in Chapter 5. If you're having shoulder trouble, use the exercises in Chapter 21.

Even though there are seven exercises, it is unlikely that in any one session you will need to do more than two. So the exercise program is neither hard nor time-consuming.

The purpose of the neck exercises is to eliminate pain and, where possible, restore normal function; that is, to regain full mobility in the neck or as much movement as possible under the given circumstances. When you are exercising for pain relief, you should move to the edge of the pain or just into the pain, then release the pressure and return to the starting position. But when you are exercising for stiffness, the exercises can be made more effective by using your hands to gently but firmly apply overpressure (more pressure than you can apply through unassisted movement of the head or neck) in order to obtain the maximum amount of movement. After doing the exercises, you should always correct your posture and then maintain the correct posture. Once you no longer have neck pain, good postural habits will be essential to prevent the recurrence of neck problems.

In order to determine whether the exercise program in this chapter is right for you, it is very important that you observe closely any changes in the location of the pain. You may notice that, as a result of the exercises, the pain, originally felt on one side of the spine, across the shoulders, or down the arm, moves toward the center of your neck. In other words, your pain localizes or centralizes. *As with back pain, centralization of neck pain (Fig. 12.1) that takes*

Figure 12.1: The progressive centralization of pain as a result of the McKenzie exercise program

place as you exercise is a good sign. If your pain moves from areas farther away from the neck—that is, if it moves from areas in which it usually is felt—and toward the midline of the spine, that means you are exercising correctly and that the McKenzie exercise program is the right one for you.

If your neck pain is so intense that you can move your head only with difficulty and cannot find a position that permits you to lie in bed comfortably, your approach to the exercises should be especially cautious and unhurried.

On beginning any of the exercises, you may notice an increase in pain. *This initial pain increase is common and can be expected.* As you continue to practice the exercises, the pain should quickly diminish, at least to the level you experienced before the exercises. Usually this occurs during the first exercise session. This should then be followed by centralization of pain.

Once the pain no longer spreads outward and it is felt only at the midline, the intensity of pain will decrease rapidly over a period of two to three days. In a further two to three days your pain should disappear entirely.

Specifically, pain can improve in many ways:

- It can become less intense.
- It can become less frequent.
- You can sustain activity longer before the pain occurs.
- You can move farther before pain begins.
- Constant pain can be replaced by intermittent pain.
- Pain can centralize. (This not only provides for a more comfortable type of pain but predicts a good outcome through the McKenzie exercises.)

If, however, following an initial increase in pain, the pain continues to increase or spreads to places farther away from the spine, immediately stop exercising. Seek advice from a health professional. In other words, do not continue with any of the exercises if your symptoms are much worse immediately after exercising and remain worse the next day. Also stop the exercises if, during exercise, you experience symptoms in the arm below the elbow for the first time or if you experience a worsening in symptoms below the elbow that you already had.

If you need advice from a health professional, ideally you will consult a credentialed member or associate of the McKenzie Institute. To obtain the names of these practitioners, see Appendix A at the back of this book.

If your symptoms have been present more or less continuously for many weeks or months, you should not expect to be pain free in two or three days. The response will be slower than if your symptoms were recent, but if you are doing the correct exercises, it will be only a matter of ten to fourteen days before the pain subsides. If you are lucky, it will be faster than that.

When learning the exercises, you should adopt the sitting position. Once you fully master them, you may exercise while sitting or standing, whichever you prefer.

Nevertheless, if the pain is too acute for you to tolerate the exercises while sitting, you may need to begin exercising while lying down. In the lying position, the pain will be reduced, because the head and neck are better supported and the compressive forces on the spine are considerably less. If you are age sixty or older, it is also advisable to begin exercising while lying down. People of older age groups occasionally experience dizziness or light-headedness when performing extension exercises involving the head (of the seven exercises in this chapter, Neck Exercises 1 through 6 all involve extension). If symptoms such as these persist, stop the exercises and seek advice from a health professional. On the other hand, when the initial attempts at extension exercises in lying do not have any ill effects, you can safely proceed to exercising while sitting.

If, due to a medical problem, it is difficult or not advisable for you to lie flat, you should restrict yourself to exercising in the sitting position. People who are over sixty and who also should not lie flat should attempt the exercises from a sitting position but should be cautious when first trying them. The first time they try the exercise, they should have another person at their side to assist in the event of dizziness or light-headedness.

When beginning this exercise program, you should stop any other exercises that you may have been shown by a health professional. You should also temporarily stop any workout or sports activities. If you want to continue with exercises other than those described in this book, you should wait until your pain has completely subsided. If you are intent on returning to sports before your pain has subsided, you must nonetheless avoid all contact sports. As for noncontact sports, you can gently attempt a return to them; if, after a short trial, your pain is worse, you must discontinue even noncontact sports until your pain has completely subsided.

Once you have started this exercise program, new pains may develop, because you are performing movements your body is not used to. The new pains are different from your original pain and are usually felt in areas of the neck and shoulder girdle that were not previously affected. But, provided you continue with the exercises, these pains will wear off in three to four days.

I always suspect that if my patients do not complain of new pains, they have not been exercising adequately or they have not been putting enough effort into correcting their posture. Both new exercises and new postures are likely to cause temporary new pains.

I cannot overstress the importance of doing the exercises precisely as they are described in this book. That is, it is important to do each exercise exactly as it is described and to do the exercises in the order that is set out in this book. The failure to heed even one sentence in the description of an exercise can keep the exercise from being effective. Don't figure that you can save time by glancing at the instructions for a particular exercise or by trying to learn an exercise just by looking at the photographs that accompany it. In this way you may save a minute or two, but slow your recovery by weeks—not a good bargain.

Similarly, don't skimp. Generally, the exercises should be done six to eight times a day. If you do them once or twice a day, you may gain some benefit, but not nearly what you would gain if you did them as often as prescribed.

There are decades of clinical experience and research behind these exercises: how to do them, in what order to do them, how often to do them. I want you to benefit as much as possible from them. Don't get in the way of your own recovery!

NECK EXERCISE 1

Head Retraction in Sitting

This is the first McKenzie exercise for the *neck*. Again, if you are a *back* patient, you will find the McKenzie exercises for the back in Chapter 5. If you're having shoulder trouble, use the exercises in Chapter 21.

An exercise session is a series of repetitions of one or more exercises. Until you can do one or more of the other McKenzie neck exercises without acute pain, each time you exercise you must begin with Neck Exercise 1, followed by Neck Exercise 2.

Head retraction means pulling the head backward.

Sit on a chair or stool, look straight ahead, and allow yourself to relax completely. As you do this, your head will protrude a little (Fig. 12.2). Now you are ready to start the first and most important exercise.

Move your head slowly but steadily backward until it is pulled back as far as you can manage. As you do this, it is important to *keep your chin tucked down and in*. In other words, you must remain looking straight ahead and should not tilt the head backward as if looking up. When your head is pulled back as far as possible, you have assumed the retracted head posture (Fig. 12.3). Once you have maintained this position for a few seconds, you should relax, and automatically your head and neck will protrude again (Fig. 12.2). Each time you repeat this cycle of movements, you must make sure that the backward movement of the head and neck is performed to the *maximum possible degree*.

Figure 12.2: The relaxed position allows the head to protrude.

Figure 12.3: The retracted position

Figure 12.4: Retraction with overpressure

As with all other McKenzie Method back, neck, and shoulder exercises involving multiple movements, remember to slowly think or say the words "pressure on, pressure off" as you do the exercise. This helps you to hold each position just long enough and establishes a rhythm in which to do the exercise.

You can use overpressure to make the exercise more effective: place both hands on the chin and firmly push the head even farther back (Fig. 12.4).

CASE HISTORY: A REAL (ESTATE) STORY

Carl, forty-five, is a real estate agent in Massachusetts. Following an auto accident, he had sharp neck pain. He saw his chiropractor, and the appointments made his neck feel better but had no lasting effect.

Carl canceled all but his most critical appointments and rested at home as much as he could. One Saturday, his mother was to host a birthday party for Carl's younger brother, Dave. Carl didn't want to be the only absentee, so, with difficulty, he got himself to the restaurant where the party was being held. Dave told him how he himself had been helped by the McKenzie neck exercises. Even so, both Dave and Carl feared that Carl's pain was so sharp that it wouldn't respond to the exercises.

Nonetheless, the day after the party, Dave sent Carl a copy of the McKenzie neck exercises. Carl tried several of them. To his amazement, he found that just one of them—Neck Exercise 1, Head Retraction in Sitting—gave him dramatic relief in just one session.

He continued with Exercise 1, added Exercise 2, Neck Extension in Sitting, and paid careful attention to his posture. Within one week he was 80 percent better and two weeks later he was pain free. His symptoms did not return.

This exercise is used mainly in the *treatment* of neck pain, as opposed to its *prevention*. When used in the *treatment* of neck pain, the exercise should be repeated ten times per session, and the sessions should be spread evenly six to eight times throughout the day. This means you should repeat the sessions about every two hours. If you experience acute pain on attempting this exercise, you must replace it with Neck Exercise 3, Head Retraction in Lying. When used in the *prevention* of neck pain, the exercise should be repeated five or six times as many times a day as required. That is, if you find you can prevent neck pain by performing two sessions of this exercise, then do two sessions a day, and if you can prevent it only by doing ten sessions a day, do ten.

NECK EXERCISE 2

Neck Extension in Sitting

Extension means bending backward.

This exercise should always follow Neck Exercise 1. Remain seated, repeat Exercise 1 a few times, then hold your head in the retracted position (Fig. 12.5). Now you are ready to start Exercise 2.

CASE HISTORY: WATCH OUT FOR FIVE-YEAR-OLDS

Ronnie, a Californian, plays lead guitar in a well-known rock band. He is fifty-two. Due to an auto accident whiplash injury, he had a recurring neck condition that most of the time caused him no pain. Two physical therapists who had treated him had shown him the McKenzie exercises. One evening he was standing near his five-year-old daughter. She expressed her affection by giving him a hug. Unfortunately, she chose to do this by jumping up and grabbing him around the neck, briefly suspending her forty-five pounds from that fragile body part.

The guitar player had immediate pain. That evening he tried the McKenzie exercises as he remembered them, plus rest, ibuprofen, and ice. All helped some, none helped enough.

The next day he went to his office, where he had a copy of the McKenzie exercises. He realized that he had forgotten all about Neck Exercise 2, Neck Extension in Sitting. He marveled at how the small point of moving the head left and right about a half inch from the midline permitted him to make his head go back farther and farther.

After the first session of this exercise, Ronnie's pain was 70 percent better. He had improved so much that he could return to all his normal activities. The next session brought the improvement to about 80 percent. The next day, he was about 90 percent better. All due to one exercise and to doing it *exactly* as McKenzie instructs patients to do it. Within two weeks, his symptoms were entirely gone.

Figure 12.5: The retracted position

Figure 12.6: Lift your chin up and tilt your head backward, as if you were looking up at the sky.

Figures 12.7a–12.7b: With your head tilted as far back as possible, repeatedly turn your nose just half an inch to the right and then to the left of the midline.

Lift your chin up and tilt your head backward, as if you were looking up at the sky (Fig. 12.6). As you do this, *do not allow your neck to move forward*. With your head tilted back as far as possible, repeatedly turn your nose just a half inch (about two centimeters) to the right and then to the left of the midline (Figs. 12.7a and 12.7b), all the time attempting to move your head and neck even farther backward. Once you have done this for a few seconds, return your head to the starting position. Again, each time you repeat this cycle of movements, make sure your neck is extended as far as possible.

This exercise can be used in both the treatment and the prevention of neck pain. Neck Exercise 2 is to be performed ten times per session, and the sessions should be spread evenly six to eight times throughout the day. If your pain is too acute to tolerate Exercise 2, you should replace it with Neck Exercise 3, Head Retraction in Lying.

Once you are fully practiced in Neck Exercises 1 and 2 separately from one another, you can combine these two exercises successfully into one exercise.

NECK EXERCISE 3

Head Retraction in Lying

Lie on a bed. Lie faceup, with your head at a free-standing edge of the bed rather than next to any headboard. For example, lie across a double bed or with your head at the foot of a single bed that has no footboard. Rest your head and shoulders flat on the bed and do not use a pillow (Fig. 12.8). Now you are ready to start Neck Exercise 3.

Using your head alone, not your hands, push the back of your head into the mattress and at the same time pull in your chin (Fig. 12.9). The overall effect should be that your head and neck move backward as far as possible while you keep facing the ceiling. Once you have maintained this position for a few seconds,

Figure 12.8: Rest your head and shoulders flat on the bed.

relax. Automatically, your head and neck will return to the starting position (Fig. 12.8). Each time you repeat this cycle of movements, make sure that the backward movement of your head and neck is carried out to the maximum possible degree.

This exercise is used mainly in the treatment of acute neck pain. It is used mostly by people who have gained no benefit from exercises done in the sitting or standing position. It is an effective exercise, but not as demanding as most of the others. When you have completed ten head retractions, you must evaluate the effects of this exercise on your pain. If the pain has centralized or decreased in intensity, you can safely continue this procedure. In this case you should repeat the exercise ten times per session and spread the sessions evenly six to eight times throughout the day or night. (Since you already are in bed at night, night is a good time to repeat this exercise.)

Figure 12.9: Push the back of your head into the mattress and at the same time pull in your chin.

If, however, the pain has increased considerably or extends farther away from the spine, or if you have developed "pins and needles" or numbness in the fingers, you must stop the exercise and seek advice from a health professional. To locate a practitioner who is a credentialed member or associate of the McKenzie Institute, see Appendix A of this book.

NECK EXERCISE 4

Neck Extension in Lying

This exercise should always follow Neck Exercise 3. You must again lie on the bed, faceup. Before you can start Neck Exercise 4, you must support your

Figure 12.10: Place one hand under your head and extend your head, your neck, and the top of your shoulders over the edge of the bed.

Figure 12.11: While supporting your head, lower it slowly toward the floor.

head by placing one hand under it. Now move up along the bed until your head, your neck, and the top of your shoulders are extended over the edge (Fig. 12.10).

While continuing to support your head with your hand, lower your head slowly toward the floor (Fig. 12.11). Now, gradually remove your hand (Fig. 12.12) and bring your head and neck as far backward as you can, so that

Figure 12.12: Gradually remove your hand and bring your head and neck as far backward as you can.

Figure 12.13: Repeatedly turn your nose just half an inch to the right and then to the left of the midline.

you can see as much as possible of the floor directly under you. In this position, repeatedly turn your nose just a half inch (about two centimeters) to the right and then to the left of the midline (Fig. 12.13), all the time attempting to move your head and neck farther backward. Once you have reached the maximum amount of extension, try to relax in this position for two to three seconds.

In order to return to the resting position, first place one hand behind your head, then help your head back to the horizontal position and move your body down along the bed until your head is lying fully on the bed again. It is important that, following this exercise, *you do not get up from the bed immediately* but instead you rest for a few minutes with your head flat on the bed. *Do not use a pillow.*

As with Neck Exercise 3, this exercise is used mainly in the treatment of acute neck pain. Also as with Exercise 3, it is effective, yet not as demanding as most of the others. Until the acute symptoms have subsided, Neck Exercise 4 is to follow Exercise 3, and Exercise 4 should be done only once per session. Once you no longer have acute pains, Exercises 3 and 4 should be replaced by Exercises 1 and 2. By now you will have noticed that, except for the position in which they are performed, Exercises 3 and 4 are really the same as Exercises 1 and 2.

NECK EXERCISE 5

Side Bending of the Neck

Sit on a chair. Repeat Neck Exercise 1 a few times, then hold your head in the retracted position (Fig. 12.14). Now you are ready to start Neck Exercise 5.

Bend your neck sideways and move your head toward the side on which you feel most of the pain. Do not allow the head to turn (Fig. 12.15). In other words, keep looking straight ahead and bring your ear—*not your nose*—close to your shoulder. It is important that you *keep the head well retracted as you do this. The exercise can be made more effective by using the hand of the painful side, placing it over the top of your head, and gently but firmly pulling your head even farther toward the painful side (Fig. 12.16).*

Figure 12.14: The retracted position

Figure 12.15: Bend your neck sideways and move your head toward the side on which you feel most of the pain.

Figure 12.16: Gently but firmly pull your head even farther toward the painful side.

Once you have maintained this position for a few seconds, return your head to the starting position.

This exercise is used specifically for the treatment of pain felt only to one side or pain felt much more to one side than the other. Until your symptoms have centralized, Neck Exercise 5 is to be repeated ten times per session and the sessions are to be spread evenly six to eight times throughout the day.

NECK EXERCISE 6

Neck Rotation

In this book, *rotation* means turning to the right and left.

Sit on a chair, repeat Neck Exercise 1 a few times, then hold your head in the retracted position (Fig. 12.17). Now you are ready to start Neck Exercise 6.

Turn your head far to the right and then far to the left, as though you were about to cross a street (Fig. 12.18). As you do this, it is important that you *keep the head well retracted*. If you experience more pain as you turn to one side

Figure 12.17: The retracted position

Figure 12.18: Turn your head far to the right and then far to the left.

than to the other, continue the exercise by rotating only to the *more* painful side. As you repeatedly turn to that side, the pain should gradually centralize or decrease.

CASE HISTORY: IF AT FIRST YOU DON'T SUCCEED . . .

Larry, a forty-eight-year-old public interest lawyer in Washington, D.C., was a neck sufferer who at first did not benefit much from the exercises but then took a second look and found what he needed.

He had suffered a whiplash injury when he was waiting to turn left at an intersection and a driver behind him was talking to her child instead of watching the road. Larry's pain was chiefly on the right side, including not just the neck but the shoulder and upper back. Sometimes he had tingling in the fingers of his right hand. He saw his family doctor, then an orthopedist, and then a physical therapist for six months. He improved, but only slowly. Advil helped, but did nothing for the underlying cause of the pain.

Then Larry got a copy of the McKenzie exercises for the neck. Naturally enough, he started out with Neck Exercise 1, Head Retraction in Sitting, and Neck Exercise 2, Neck Extension in Sitting. These gave him only minor relief. But then he tried Neck Exercise 5, Side Bending of the Neck, which is indicated specifically for people with pain exclusively on one side or much more on one side than the other.

He improved rapidly. The first time he did the exercises, the pain centralized in the midline, and Larry found the pain much more tolerable there than when it was on the right side. At the same time, the pain declined markedly. Within a week, the pain was no longer a problem in his life, and in about a month his symptoms had vanished entirely.

But if the pain increases and fails to centralize, continue the exercise by rotating only to the *less* painful side.

Once you have the same amount of pain when turning to either side, or you have no pain when turning to either side, continue the exercise by rotating to both sides.

The exercise can be made more effective by using both hands to gently but firmly push your head even farther into rotation (Figs. 12.19a and 12.19b). Once you have maintained the position of maximum rotation for a few seconds, return your head to the starting position.

This exercise can be used in the treatment of neck pain as well as for its prevention. When used in the *treatment* of pain or stiffness of the neck, the exercise is to be performed ten times per session, and the sessions are to be spread evenly six to eight times throughout the day. Whether or not centralization or a decrease in pain has taken place, *Neck Exercise 6 must always be followed by Neck Exercises 1 and 2.* When used in the *prevention* of neck problems, the exercise should be repeated five or six times every two or three days or as often as required.

NECK EXERCISE 7

Neck Flexion in Sitting

Flexion means bending forward.

Sit on a chair, look straight ahead, and allow yourself to relax completely (Fig. 12.20). Now you are ready to start Neck Exercise 7.

Drop your head forward and let it rest with your chin as close as possible to your chest (Fig. 12.21). Place your hands behind the back of your head and interlock your fingers (Fig. 12.22). Now let your arms relax so that your elbows point down toward the floor. In this position, the weight of your arms will pull your head down farther and bring your chin closer to your chest (Fig. 12.23).

This exercise can be made more effective by using your hands to gently but firmly pull your head onto your chest. Once you have maintained the position of maximum neck flexion for a few seconds, return your head to the starting position.

This exercise is used mainly for the treatment of *headaches*, but it can also be applied to resolve residual neck pain or stiffness once the acute symptoms have subsided. In both cases, it should be repeated only two or three times per session, and the sessions should be spread evenly six to eight times throughout the day.

When used in the treatment of headaches, Neck Exercise 7 should be performed in conjunction with Neck Exercise 1. For more on this, see the section titled "When You Have Headaches" in Chapter 13. When used in the treatment of neck pain or stiffness, Neck Exercise 7 must always be followed by Neck Exercises 1 and 2.

Figures 12.19a–12.19b: Use both hands and gently but firmly push your head even farther into rotation.

Figure 12.20: Sit on a chair, look straight ahead, and allow yourself to relax completely.

Figure 12.21: Drop your head forward and let it rest with your chin as close as possible to your chest.

Figure 12.22: Place your hands behind the back of your head and interlock your fingers.

Figure 12.23: Let your arms relax so the elbows point down toward the floor.

CASE HISTORY: CONVINCING THE DOCS

Catherine lives in Arkansas. She is forty years old and works as a receptionist in the office of several physicians. Before starting the McKenzie program, she had for four months suffered from neck pain, headaches, and difficulty in swallowing. Two months before the symptoms began, the medical office had been remodeled and she had been given a new phone system and a different desk.

Catherine's McKenzie-certified physical therapist concluded that Catherine had cervical disc inflammation resulting from her posture while talking on the phone and while typing on a computer keyboard; both these postures had changed because of the remodeling of the office.

The physical therapist prescribed Neck Exercise 7, Neck Flexion in Sitting. Doctors had attributed her swallowing difficulties to allergies, but with Neck Exercise 7, this symptom immediately disappeared. Before trying Exercise 7, Catherine described her pain as a 5 on a scale of 0 to 10, but after doing Exercise 7 for the first time, she said her pain had declined to a 1.

Catherine visited the physical therapist four times over two weeks and threw away her allergy medications. Over this period, her neck pain and headaches resolved completely. She remained pain free. She was not the only one impressed by the effects of the McKenzie program: after she reported her results to the people at her office, the physicians and her coworkers also became believers in the McKenzie Method.

13 WHEN TO DO THE NECK EXERCISES

You should seek advice from your doctor if your neck pain is of such severity that it is impossible to perform these exercises (or other exercises in this book) or your pain is becoming intolerable.

WHEN YOU ARE IN SIGNIFICANT PAIN

When your neck pain is very acute, you may still be able to get out of bed, although probably with difficulty. But certain movements will be impossible and often you will not be able to find a comfortable position in which to sit or work. But even if you are in acute pain, you should always attempt to begin with Neck Exercise 1. Many people find that this exercise gives substantial relief from pain and that they do not have to start with the exercises that involve lying on a bed (Neck Exercises 3 and 4).

As soon as possible, even on the first day, you should add Neck Exercise 2. You should continue Exercises 1 and 2 until you feel considerably better. Once you no longer have acute pain, you should follow the exercise program as outlined in this chapter under the heading "When Acute Pain Has Subsided."

If you have done three or four sessions of Exercise 1, spread over a period of fifteen minutes, and the pain remains too acute to tolerate that exercise, you should stop it and replace it with Neck Exercise 3. Your symptoms should gradually decrease and centralize so that there is some improvement by the time you have completed a few sessions. Neck Exercise 4 should be added as soon as you have become well practiced in Exercise 3 and your symptoms have improved to some extent, or when Exercise 3 is no longer bringing you any improvement.

When the person with neck pain should introduce Exercise 4 varies from person to person, but the sooner you can do this, the better. It is important that you carefully watch the pain pattern. You are exercising correctly if within a few days the pain moves toward the base or the center of the neck and decreases. In time the pain should disappear entirely and be replaced by a feeling of strain or stiffness, a feeling that is more tolerable.

When you have improved significantly—usually two to three days after you began the exercises that involve lying on a bed, possibly earlier—you may gradually reduce the number of sessions of Neck Exercises 3 and 4. As you do this, you should gradually introduce Exercises 1 and 2 and then gradually increase these two exercises.

In another few days you will be doing only exercises in sitting (instead of exercises done while lying on a bed), and you will find that they give you the same pain relief as you previously obtained by performing the movements while on a bed. At this stage, the periods when you are completely free of pain will be occurring more frequently and beginning to last longer.

Again, once you feel considerably better and no longer have acute pain, you should continue the exercise program as outlined below, under the heading "When Acute Pain Has Subsided."

WHEN YOU GET NO RESPONSE OR BENEFIT

When pain is felt only to one side of the spine or much more to one side than the other, the neck exercises recommended so far sometimes fail to bring relief. If this is the case, you should begin with Neck Exercise 5. Whether or not centralization or a decrease in pain has taken place, Exercise 5 must always be followed by Neck Exercises 1 and 2. After two or three days of practice, you may notice that the pain is distributed more evenly across the spine or it has centralized. Once either of these events has occurred, you may gradually reduce Exercise 5.

When you are considerably better—the acute pain has subsided and the pain has fully centralized—you should continue with the exercise program as outlined next.

WHEN ACUTE PAIN HAS SUBSIDED

Once the acute pain has passed, you may still feel some pain or stiffness when you move in certain ways. You will notice this most clearly when you turn your neck to one side or the other or when you bend your head and neck forward in order to look down. It is likely that at this stage, healing of overstretched or damaged soft tissues has taken place. Now you must ensure that the elasticity of these soft tissues and the flexibility of your spine as a whole are restored without causing you further damage.

If you have pain on turning your head to the right or left, you should practice Neck Exercise 6. If you have pain on bending your head forward, you need to practice Neck Exercise 7. Each time you repeat an exercise, you must move to the edge of the pain and then release the pressure. The pain should disappear entirely over a period of two to three weeks. Each session of Exercises 6 and 7 should always be concluded with a few repetitions of Neck Exercises 1 and 2.

If you feel stiffness but no pain in these exercises, you should do the same exercises but apply overpressure with your hands at the end of each movement. By exercising in this way, you achieve the maximum possible movement. In three to six weeks you should be able to restore normal function.

Once you are completely symptom free, and you have no pain or stiffness, you should follow the guidelines outlined next to prevent recurrence of neck problems.

WHEN YOU HAVE NO PAIN OR STIFFNESS

Many people with neck problems have lengthy spells in which they experience little or no pain. If, in the past or recently, you have had one or more episodes of neck pain, you should start the exercise program even though at the moment you may be pain free. Nevertheless, in this situation it is not necessary to do all the exercises you would do if you were in pain or to do the exercises every two hours.

To prevent recurrence of neck problems, you should do Neck Exercise 6, followed by Neck Exercises 1 and 2. You should do these regularly, preferably in the morning and at night. Furthermore, whenever you feel minor strain developing during work or while sitting, you should do Exercises 1 and 2. It is even more important that you watch your posture at all times and never again let postural stresses cause you neck pain.

These exercises will have very little or no effect if you constantly fall back into poor posture. It may be necessary to exercise in the manner described above for the rest of your life, but it is essential that you develop and maintain good postural habits.

As it takes only one minute to perform one session of Neck Exercise 6 and another minute to combine Exercises 1 and 2 and repeat them ten times, lack of time should never be used as an excuse for not doing the exercises.

WHEN YOU HAVE A RECURRENCE

At the first sign of recurrence of neck pain, you should immediately perform Neck Exercises 1 and 2. If your pain already is too acute to tolerate these exercises, or if they fail to reduce your pain, you must quickly introduce Exercises 3 and 4. If you have one-sided symptoms that do not centralize with any of these exercises, you should start with Exercise 5. Again, you must pay extra attention to your posture, regularly perform postural correction, and maintain the correct posture as much as you can.

WHEN YOU HAVE HEADACHES

Headaches often can be relieved by some of the recommended exercises, usually Neck Exercises 1 and 7. Unless your neck pain is severe, it will not do any harm to perform these exercises for a couple of days in order to find out whether you benefit from them or not. In the first three days, you should perform Exercise 1, Head Retraction in Sitting, at regular intervals and whenever you feel a headache is developing. If this reduces your headaches but does not eliminate them, you should add Exercise 7, Neck Flexion in Sitting. Exercise 7 is particularly effective in relieving headaches that spread over the top of your head to above or behind the eyes. You may even be able to *prevent* such headaches by performing this exercise as soon as you feel minor strain building up.

In case your headaches are not relieved by these two exercises, for the next three days you should do Exercise 4, Neck Extension in Lying, followed by Exercises 1 and 2 and postural correction. As your symptoms improve, you may gradually stop Exercise 4 but you must continue Exercises 1 and 2.

If you are unable to influence your headaches with any of the exercises or if your headaches become much worse while performing them and remain worse over the next day, you should stop doing them and seek advice from a health professional. A credentialed member or associate of the McKenzie Institute would be especially well qualified to assist you. To obtain the names of these practitioners, see Appendix A at the back of this book.

14 INSTRUCTIONS FOR PEOPLE WITH ACUTE NECK PAIN

CHANCES ARE, IF YOU HAVE NECK PAIN YOU CAN USE THIS BOOK IMME-
diately. Nevertheless, if you have developed neck pain for the first time and it
is no better ten days after onset, do not use this book until you have consulted
your doctor. Likewise, if you have complications to your neck problems, do not
use this book until you have consulted your doctor. Examples of complications
are severe, stabbing pains; your head being pulled off center; or severe, continuing headaches.

Keep your head up at all times. When you allow the head to droop while
you are engaged in activities such as working at a desk, reading, knitting, or
sewing, you place further strains on the already overstretched or injured tissues. It is essential to maintain good posture.

Do not roll your head around. Avoid quick movements, especially turning
the head quickly.

Avoid the positions and movements that caused your problems in the first
place. You must allow some time for healing to take place.

Do not sleep with more pillows than necessary. If you are comfortable
with one pillow, then use only one. The contents of the pillow should be adjustable so that the pillow provides proper support for your neck.

If you remain uncomfortable while sleeping or attempting to sleep, you may benefit by placing a cervical roll inside your pillowcase.

Do not sleep facedown, as this places great strain on the neck.

Do not lie in the bath for any length of time, as this bends your head and neck forward excessively.

Carefully start the self-treatment exercises. Remember, an initial increase in pain can be expected when beginning any of the exercises. This pain should decrease or centralize, or both, as you repeat the movements.

(In the event that you have a sudden onset of acute neck pain and need a quick summary of what to do, consult Chapter 16, "Panic Pages for the Neck.")

ALTERNATIVES TO THE MCKENZIE NECK EXERCISES

Health professionals and others offer many ways to treat neck pain. In Chapter 9, I deal with many of these, regarding how they relate to back pain. I also deal with back pain in the community. Therefore I refer you to Chapter 9.

With few exceptions, I would simply substitute the word "neck" or the word "shoulder" for "back" and "lower back" and then leave Chapter 9 as is. One exception is that bed rest, while appropriate in a small minority of cases of back pain, is appropriate even more rarely for neck or shoulder. While a bed may be the only practical way to support a severely painful back, a much smaller device supports the neck fairly well in those cases where the neck should be treated almost exclusively by resting it. In these rare cases you should consult a doctor and then, if he or she recommends doing so, give your neck a rest by using a soft foam rubber cervical collar for short periods. Continue to use it if it immediately reduces your discomfort, but do not use it for more than three or four weeks.

Regarding neck pain in the community, a difference between Chapter 9 and what I would say about the neck is that in Western countries, approximately 40 percent will at one time suffer a severe neck pain episode (not the 80 percent in the case of the back). I am unaware of any study on the percentage for the shoulder.

Because the neck and shoulder depend on good back posture, the neck and shoulder patient, just like the back patient, should seek good furniture and good seating in transit situations and should complain when these are not available. Similarly, it is important not only for the back but for the neck and shoulders that school physical education instructors teach posture and the consequences of bad posture. Again, for information on the McKenzie Institute's posture correction video, which is available to schools, please see Appendix A.

15 PANIC PAGES FOR THE BACK

IN CASE OF A SUDDEN ONSET OF ACUTE BACK PAIN, OBSERVE THE FOL-lowing precautions. Then, if you can use this book, proceed with the instructions.

PRECAUTIONS

If you have unusual complications, do not use this book or this chapter until you have consulted your doctor, physical therapist, or chiropractor. Examples of complications include constant pain that travels down your leg all the way to the foot, numbness or weak muscles, or a general sense of feeling unwell.

Likewise, if you have developed severe back pain for the first time and it is no better ten days after onset, do not use this book or this chapter until you have consulted your doctor, physical therapist, or chiropractor.

Figure 15.1: Exercise 1

Figure 15.2: Exercise 2

Figure 15.3: Exercise 3

INSTRUCTIONS

1. Immediately lie facedown.

If this is impossible because of pain intensity, go to bed. Attempt these exercises the next day.

2. When resting in bed, use a rolled towel or a lumbar night roll around your waist.

3. Perform Back Exercises 1, 2, and 3 (Figs. 15.1–3). Every two hours, perform Exercises 1 and 2 once and Exercise 3 ten times. Perform Exercise 1 for two to three minutes, Exercise 2 for two to three minutes, and Exercise 3 ten times, which will take one to two minutes. (For details on all the McKenzie back exercises, see Chapter 5.)

4. If the pain is more to one side and not decreasing: while lying facedown, move hips away from the painful side and do Back Exercises 2 and 3.

5. Rest as much as possible, correctly supported.

6. Do not bend forward for three to four days.

7. Sit perfectly at all times—use a lumbar roll.

16 PANIC PAGES FOR THE NECK

IN CASE OF A SUDDEN ONSET OF ACUTE NECK PAIN, OBSERVE THE FOL-lowing precautions. Then, if you can use this book, proceed with the instructions.

PRECAUTIONS

If you have developed neck pain for the first time and it is no better ten days after onset, do not use this book or this chapter until you have consulted your doctor.

Likewise, if you have complications to your neck problems, do not use this book or this chapter until you have consulted your doctor. Examples of complications are severe, stabbing pains; your head being pulled off center; or severe, continuing headaches.

Figure 16.1: Exercise 3

Figure 16.2: Exercise 4

Figure 16.3: Exercise 5

INSTRUCTIONS

1. Do not rest in bed. Keep your head as still as possible. Avoid all painful movements.
2. When sitting, use a lumbar roll to maintain a safe posture.
3. Do not bend the neck forward, roll the head around, or make quick movements of the head or neck.
4. First attempt Neck Exercise 1, Head Retraction in Sitting. If Exercise 1 provides some relief, add Neck Exercise 2, Neck Extension in Sitting. If, however, Exercise 1 has no effect or it makes your symptoms worse, go immediately to Neck Exercises 3 and 4 (Figs. 16.1 and 16.2), performing them every two hours. Do Exercise 3 ten times every two hours; do Exercise 4 once every two hours. (For details on all the McKenzie neck exercises, see Chapter 12.)
5. When pain is more to one side and not responding to Neck Exercise 1, 2, 3, or 4, do Exercise 5 (Fig. 16.3), followed by Exercises 1 and 2. Do Exercises 5, 1, and 2 ten times every two hours.

17 SHOULDER PROBLEMS

AT SOME TIME DURING OUR LIVES MANY OF US SUFFER FROM PAIN OR stiffness in the region of the shoulder, or pain arising from the shoulder that is felt in the upper arm. It is one of the most common problems affecting the joints and muscles, after back pain and neck pain.

What's more, these problems frequently persist or recur, with about 50 percent of people still having problems a year after the onset of their shoulder pain. The American Academy of Orthopaedic Surgeons reports that more than 4 million people in the United States seek medical attention each year for shoulder pain, and it accounts for 1.5 million visits to orthopedic surgeons.

Shoulder problems are often referred to in different ways, including tendonitis, rotator cuff strain or tear, impingement syndrome, frozen shoulder, capsulitis, or arthritis. But even health professionals often have difficulty in identifying a specific source of the pain due to the complex nature of the shoulder and its close involvement with the neck. In many cases, even the use of X-rays, ultrasound scans, and MRI scans do not give an exact picture of the site or severity of the injury or give clear guidance for treatment strategies. In fact, the emphasis is often on labeling the patient's condition, without doing much to resolve it.

Shoulder pain can be felt in a variety of ways. There may be days or times in the day when no pain is felt. The symptoms may appear for no apparent reason, and just as mysteriously they disappear. At other times the symptoms may occur only with specific movements of the arm, such as getting dressed, reaching up into a cupboard, or reaching into the back pocket of your trousers. These aches and pains may also occur constantly—that is, pain to some degree is felt at all times throughout the day. It is also common for shoulder pain to regularly disturb sleep. People who have pain all the time are frequently forced to take medication and sometimes have to stop work. The pain simply makes their lives miserable, and they have to reduce their activities in order to keep the discomfort at a moderate level. Shoulder problems can thus significantly affect quality of life. If you have problems of this nature, you may have already discovered that the symptoms can sometimes last for months or even years. You may have found that some treatments can decrease or stop your pain temporarily, but the pain returns later to affect you once again. You may be reading this book because you have persistent pain that has not disappeared, despite the fact that you may have received many types of treatments.

Common treatments for shoulder pain are medications, injections, acupuncture, or electrical modalities such as ultrasound, TENS (transcutaneous electrical nerve stimulation), and interferential therapy. However, while some of these treatments may appear to give short-term benefit, none have strong evidence that they provide effective long-term relief from pain and loss of function.

Figure 17.1: Raising the arms in a construction job can contribute to shoulder problems.

You may also have been given exercises to perform and have found these to be of some benefit. However, many people do not realize that stretching and strengthening your shoulder alone does not automatically give you relief from shoulder pain. "Doing your exercises" is only part of the solution, and what we seldom consider are the positions we hold our arms in the rest of the time.

It is important to realize that the way you move your arm and the sustained raised arm position or postures you adopt during manual occupations, such as building (Fig. 17.1) or hairdressing (Fig. 17.2), can significantly contribute to your shoulder problem. Similarly, it is common for people in sedentary occupations, for example, office work, to report shoulder pain related to static raised arm postures such a sitting at a computer (Fig. 17.3). Activities such as driving (Fig. 17.4), and even some sleeping postures with the arms raised (Fig. 17.5), also place a prolonged static load on the shoulder.

Figure 17.2: So can some movements of a hairdresser.

Figure 17.3: A static raised arm posture can contribute to shoulder pain.

Figure 17.4: Driving can place a prolonged static load on the shoulder.

Figure 17.5: Even some sleeping postures can cause the same problem.

Whatever the situation, you have likely realized that many of the treatments that doctors, physical therapists, and chiropractors prescribe are aimed at your current symptoms and are not directed at preventing future problems. Time and again you may have to seek assistance to get relief from your shoulder pain. Imagine how good it would be if you were able to apply treatment to yourself whenever pain arose. Better still, imagine how good it would be if you were able to apply a system of treatment to yourself that would prevent a recurrence or reduce the intensity of the pain.

It has been shown repeatedly that people require a rational explanation for their problems. They need education in the postures, activities, and exercises that allow them to remain free of disabling symptoms. They need advice on how to avoid the detrimental forces encountered in daily living and how to apply beneficial strategies. All of these things are found in this book.

One of the main points of this book is that the management of your back, neck, and shoulder pain is your responsibility. If, for some reason or other, you have developed shoulder problems, then you must learn how to deal with the present symptoms and how to prevent or limit future problems. Self-treatment will be more effective in the long-term management of your shoulder pain than any other form of treatment because you can self-treat multiple times a day. It is the least expensive treatment and safer than receiving treatment from other people. Self-management gives you the tools to stay better.

WHO CAN PERFORM SELF-TREATMENT?

The majority of people will benefit from the advice given in this book, which is designed for those people with straightforward recurring mechanical problems. Nearly everyone can do the shoulder exercise program, provided the recommended precautions are taken as described later in this chapter.

However, in any of the following situations *do not begin the exercise program* without first consulting your doctor or physical therapist:

- If you have associated neck or upper back pain (see "Diagnosing Your Problem," below).
- If you have severe pain in the arm below the elbow and experience

sensations of weakness, numbness, or "pins and needles" in the hand and fingers.

- If you have suddenly developed shoulder problems following a recent severe accident, such as a heavy fall onto an outstretched arm, resulting in a major loss of movement, or visible bruising.
- If you are generally feeling unwell in conjunction with your shoulder pain.
- If you have a previous history of cancer or a tumor.
- If you develop chest pain with activity or have a history of cardiac or heart problems.
- If you have had shoulder surgery in the past six months.
- If you have a history of repeated dislocation of your shoulder or have dislocated it recently.

If you have developed shoulder pain for the first time, you must follow the instructions and guidelines over the next several pages even more carefully. If you have any doubt about your suitability for this program, we recommend you consult your doctor or physical therapist for advice and treatment and for instructions on the prevention of further shoulder problems.

Choose your therapist carefully. He or she should provide you with the information and education you require to manage your own problem. Every patient deserves to have the opportunity to learn how to manage his or her own shoulder problem, and every therapist should be obligated to provide that information. This is the essence of the McKenzie Method.

The only health care professionals fully qualified to provide the McKenzie Method are members of the McKenzie Institute International who hold the credentialing certificate or the institute's diploma in Mechanical Diagnosis and Therapy. To obtain names of these treatment providers in your area, please see Appendix A.

We recommend you carefully follow the guidelines and instructions in the rest of this chapter to assess your suitability for this program, or to establish whether you should consult a health professional first. The information provided will enable you to determine with reasonable certainty whether your shoulder is the source of your pain, and if you will benefit from the methods outlined in this book.

Once you have started the exercises, carefully watch your pain pattern.

If your pain is getting progressively worse and remains worse the following day, or if it is slowly increasing in severity and becoming intolerable, you should seek advice from your doctor or other qualified health care professional.

DIAGNOSING YOUR PROBLEM

Differentiating Neck Pain from Shoulder Pain

The shoulder has a close relationship with the neck, or cervical region of the spine, and sometimes the pain and loss of movement a person feels in his or her shoulder is actually coming from a problem in the neck. Therefore with all shoulder problems it is important to attempt to exclude the neck as the source of the pain.

The two most reliable indicators to determine whether the pain is coming from structures in the neck or the shoulder are the pain's location and its behavior.

Pain Location

The sites of pain caused by both shoulder and neck problems can be similar in some cases. Pain originating from the shoulder is usually felt on the front or outer part of the shoulder and commonly in the upper third of the arm (Fig. 17.6). It may radiate down to the elbow and in severe cases you may occasionally feel a dull ache as far down your arm as the wrist (Fig. 17.7). Affected shoulder structures do not usually cause pain to be felt above the shoulder or into the neck. Therefore, if pain is felt between the point of the shoulder and the neck, or in the region of the shoulder blade, it is unlikely to be coming from the shoulder. A shoulder problem will not give you a sensation of "pins and needles" or numbness in the hand.

On the other hand, pain originating from structures in the neck will generally cause some pain or aching at or near the base of the neck or into the shoulder blade (Fig. 17.8). However, the most pain may also be felt between the neck and shoulder. It may spread into the shoulder and upper arm and even

Figure 17.6: Pain originating in the shoulder is commonly felt in the upper third of the arm.

Figure 17.7: Pain may radiate down to the elbow and even the wrist.

Figure 17.8: Pain originating in the neck will generally cause pain at or near the base of the neck or into the shoulder blade.

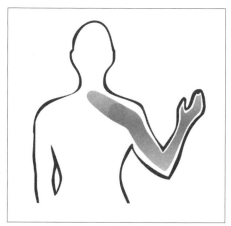

Figure 17.9: Severe pain may be felt between the neck and shoulder and may spread farther.

extend below the elbow to the wrist or hand (Fig. 17.9). Pain from a neck problem may also be associated with a sensation of "pins and needles" or numbness.

Pain Behavior

In most cases, shoulder pain that originates in the shoulder itself is produced or aggravated by moving the shoulder and arm—particularly lifting your arm to the front or side or putting your hand behind your back. But shoulder pain that originates from the neck is frequently altered by neck positions or movements.

To determine whether neck movements affect your shoulder and arm pain, we recommend that you perform the following test movements, carefully noting any change in your pain location and intensity.

If these neck movements have no effect on your shoulder or arm pain it is probable that the shoulder is the source of your pain. However, if these neck movements either produce your shoulder pain or alter the intensity or location of it, the source of your pain may be the structures in your neck, and the information in the neck section of this book may be of more relevance to you.

Test: Retraction and Extension

As your starting position, sit or stand upright with both arms relaxed by your sides. Take careful note of where you have been feeling your pain. Retract your neck (Fig. 17.10) and slowly lift your chin upward as if looking at the sky (Fig. 17.11). Hold for one or two seconds, then slowly lower it again and return to the starting position. Repeat this action of retraction with extension ten times.

Figure 17.10: Retract your neck.   **Figure 17.11:** Then slowly lift your chin as if looking at the sky.

Figure 17.12: Slowly side-bend your neck toward your painful shoulder.

Figure 17.13: Repeat the motion 10 times toward the nonpainful side.

Assess the pain's behavior according to the guidelines above. If you are still in doubt you may further test your neck movements in side bending and rotation.

Test: Side Bending

Make sure you are still sitting or standing upright with both arms relaxed by your sides, taking note again of where you have been feeling pain. This time, slowly bend your neck sideways, face forward, toward your painful shoulder (Fig. 17.12). Hold for one or two seconds, then slowly return to the starting position. Repeat this action ten times, and reassess your pain. Now repeat this movement ten times to the nonpainful side (Fig. 17.13).

Figure 17.14: Slowly rotate your head toward the painful shoulder.

Figure 17.15: Repeat, but toward the nonpainful side.

Test: Rotation

From the upright sitting or standing position as above, take note again of where you have been feeling your pain. Slowly turn your head toward the painful shoulder (Fig. 17.14). Hold for one or two seconds, then slowly return to the starting position. Repeat this action ten times, and reassess your pain. Now repeat this action ten times to the nonpainful side (Fig. 17.15).

If these neck movements have no effect on your shoulder or arm pain, it is probable that the shoulder is the source of your pain. However, if any of these repeated movements of your neck appear to either produce your shoulder pain or alter the intensity or location of it, the source of the pain is probably the structures in your neck. Therefore, we strongly recommend that you read Chapters 10 through 14 of this book, on self-treatment of neck pain.

If you still have any doubt as to whether your neck is affecting your shoulder pain, you can perform the test movements again. But this time, rather than standing or sitting with your arms relaxed by your sides, raise the arm on your painful side into a painful position, and repeat the sequence of movements as above, starting with the retraction in the first test. Relax your arm between the sequences of test movements, then return to the painful position as you attempt the next movement.

BEFORE YOU BEGIN SELF-TREATMENT

Having determined that your shoulder region is the source of your pain, we recommend you spend a further couple of minutes completing the following checklist. Answering all the questions will help you to determine whether you can treat your shoulder problem successfully without further assistance.

	YES	NO
• Are there periods in the day when you have no pain? Even ten minutes?	☐	☐
• Do you have pain only when you move your arm and shoulder?	☐	☐
• Are you generally better with your arm at your side or supported across your body?	☐	☐
• Are you generally worse during or after a prolonged period of holding your arms in a raised position such as welding, driving, hedge trimming, or painting?	☐	☐
• Is your pain produced or made worse when you lie on your affected shoulder?	☐	☐
• Is the pain confined to areas above the elbow?	☐	☐
• If you have pain in the upper or lower arm does it sometimes stop completely even though you may still have pain in the shoulder?	☐	☐
• Have you had several episodes of shoulder pain over the past months or years?	☐	☐
• Between episodes, is your shoulder free of pain?	☐	☐

• Between episodes, are you able to move your arm freely in all directions without pain? ☐ ☐

If you answered yes to all of the questions you are an ideal candidate for the self-treatment outlined in this book.

If you answered yes to five or more questions, your chances to benefit from self-treatment are good and you should commence the program.

If you answered yes to fewer than five of the questions, then some form of specialized treatment may be required and you should consult a health professional, ideally a credentialed member or associate of the McKenzie Institute. To obtain the names of these practitioners in your area, see Appendix A.

This book describes a complete system of management, and it must be followed in its entirety to ensure success. Do not turn straight to the exercise description pages; your understanding of Chapters 17 to 20 is essential.

18 THE SHOULDER AND NECK REGION

LET US LOOK AT THE SHOULDER REGION.
The shoulder joint consists of a ball-and-socket joint between the long arm bone and the shoulder blade, known as the humerus and the scapula, respectively. The shoulder joint itself is surrounded by a saclike structure called a capsule, which provides stability. In front of the shoulder region is the collarbone, the clavicle, which links the chest to the outer part of the scapula. The small joint between the scapula and clavicle is known as the acromioclavicular joint, commonly called the AC joint. Collectively the humerus, clavicle, and scapula, which are held in place by ligaments, are called the shoulder girdle, and they are attached largely by muscles to the neck, upper back, and rib cage (Fig. 18.1).

For further support and movement, the

Figure 18.1: Collectively, the humerus, clavicle, and scapula, which are held in place by the ligaments, are called the "shoulder girdle" and are attached largely by muscles to the neck, upper back, and rib cage.

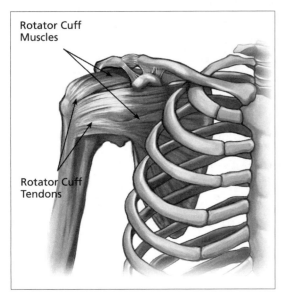

Rotator Cuff
Muscles

Rotator Cuff
Tendons

Figure 18.2: For increased support and movement, the shoulder joint relies on a small group of muscles that are collectively known as the "rotator cuff."

shoulder joint relies on a small group of muscles that are collectively known as the rotator cuff. They begin on the scapula and are attached to the top of the humerus by cordlike tissues called tendons (Fig. 18.2). When a rotator cuff muscle contracts, the tendons move with it, and movement occurs in the shoulder joint.

FUNCTIONS OF THE SHOULDER REGION

The shoulder girdle is a series of joints of which the shoulder joint is the most flexible. It is the most mobile joint in the body and allows positioning of the hand to perform a range of func-

Figure 18.3: The shoulder girdle makes us able to reach above our head . . .

Figure 18.4: . . . across our body . . .

Figure 18.5: . . . and behind our back.

tional tasks. We are able to reach above our head (Fig. 18.3), across our body (Fig. 18.4), and behind our back (Fig. 18.5) in almost 180 degrees of motion.

The design of the shoulder also allows it to focus strength and power for the performance of heavy physical tasks, such as lifting and carrying when our arms are close to the sides of the body (Fig. 18.6).

However, this strength and power capability is reduced during activities involving reaching and stretching away from the body or above the head. The flexibility of the shoulder, combined with its requirements for strength and power, makes it vulnerable to strains and overstretching from raised arm or reaching activities. If we lose this wide range of painless motion because we develop a painful shoulder it quickly has an impact on our daily life, interfering with everything from recreational activities to everyday tasks like dressing and working.

Figure 18.6: The design of the shoulder also facilitates strength and power for certain physical tasks, such as lifting or carrying when our arms are close to the side of the body.

MECHANICAL PAIN

Pain of mechanical origin occurs when a pain-sensitive structure has been placed in a position that overstretches, overloads, or compresses the surrounding ligaments, tendons, and other soft tissues. This is true for mechanical pain in any region of the body, including the shoulder. To help you understand how easily some mechanical pains can be produced, you may like to try a simple experiment. Please see the section titled "Mechanical Pain" in Chapter 2, and the photo there, where this experiment in bending a finger is described fully.

To do the experiment, bend one finger backward until you feel a strain (Fig. 18.7).

If you keep your finger in this position, you initially feel only minor discomfort, but as time passes, pain eventually develops. In some cases, pain caused by prolonged stretching may take as much as an hour

Figure 18.7: Bend your finger backward until you feel a strain.

to appear. Try the experiment once more, but now keep bending the finger past the point of strain until you feel the immediate sensation of pain. You have overstretched, and your pain warning system is telling you that to continue movement in that particular direction will cause damage. The pain warning tells you to stop overstretching to avoid damage and, when you do stop overstretching, the pain ceases immediately. No damage has occurred and the pain is gone. No lasting problems arise from this short-lived strain provided you take note of the pain warning system.

If you fail to heed the warning and keep the finger in the overstretched position, the ligaments and surrounding soft tissues that hold the joint together will eventually overstretch and tear. This tearing will result in an ache that continues even when you stop overstretching. The pain declines in intensity but continues even when the finger is at rest. The pain increases with movement performed in the wrong direction and will not cease until some healing has occurred. Healing may take several days, but this would be prolonged if every day you were to continue to apply the same strain to the finger. The same things happen when you overstretch the structures in and around your shoulder.

MECHANICAL SHOULDER PAIN

The shoulder capsule, ligaments, and the rotator cuff tendons, and other soft tissues that hold the shoulder together, can simply be overstretched, overloaded, or compressed without further damage, as in the bent finger example above. Overstretching may also be caused by a force placing a sudden, severe strain on the shoulder, for example, when mis-hitting a golf shot (Fig, 18.8), starting a sluggish lawn mower (Fig. 18.9), or taking a fall on the shoulder, elbow, or hand (Fig. 18.10). This type of stress cannot easily be avoided as it occurs unexpectedly.

However, more often overstretching or overloading is caused by postural stresses that place less severe strains on the shoulder over a longer time period, for example, when performing activities with either repeated or sustained raised arm or overhead arm positions, such as pruning, house painting, or swimming (Figs. 18.11–13). By understanding the potential for injury in

Figure 18.8: Overstretching may be caused by a force placing a sudden, severe strain on the shoulder, as in mis-hitting a golf shot . . .

Figure 18.9: . . . starting a lawnmower, . . .

Figure 18.10: . . . or falling onto the shoulder, elbow, or hand.

Figure 18.11: Overstretching or overloading can be caused by such activities as pruning . . .

Figure 18.12: . . . house painting . . .

Figure 18.13: . . . or swimming.

repeatedly performing these actions or keeping the arms raised like this for prolonged periods of time, you can learn to minimize these potentially damaging loads on your shoulders. Herein lies one of your main responsibilities in the self-treatment and prevention of shoulder pain.

TISSUE DAMAGE

Complications arise when overstretching or overloading of soft tissues around the shoulder leads to actual tissue damage. It is often thought that shoulder pain is caused by strained muscles. This is not the case. Muscles, which are the source of power and movement, can be overstretched but usually heal rapidly and seldom cause pain lasting for more than a week or two. The real problem lies in the shoulder joint tissues and the rotator cuff tendons, which are readily injured from overstretching or overloading.

If damaged, these structures undergo a healing process that may result in an incomplete repair, and thus they become less elastic and weakened. Once soft tissues are damaged, pain is felt until healing is complete and function is fully restored. We used to believe this pain was caused by chronic inflammation of these structures, and treatment was aimed at decreasing this inflammation with medication, injections, or electrotherapy. However, we now understand that the solution for these pain-sensitive structures is to remodel the tissue by gradually applying progressive forces. Unless appropriate exercises are performed to gradually stretch and strengthen these structures and restore their normal flexibility and strength, they may become a continuous source of shoulder pain.

It is also important that during this repair phase you avoid movements or sustained arm positions that disrupt the recovery process. The failure of the tissues to fully recover will result in ongoing pain and a loss of shoulder movement in some directions, along with a reduced ability to return to your usual work or daily activities.

19 COMMON CAUSES OF SHOULDER PAIN

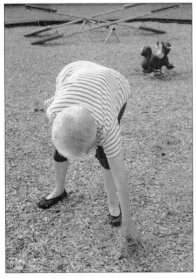

Figure 19.1: Shoulder structures may be injured and even torn when we wrench our shoulder performing a forceful lifting or pulling action, like pulling a plant out of the ground . . .

AS MENTIONED IN CHAPTER 18 THERE ARE TWO MAIN structures within the shoulder region that give rise to shoulder pain—the capsule and ligaments of the shoulder joint itself, and the surrounding rotator cuff tendons. These structures may be injured, and sometimes even torn, when we wrench our shoulder performing a forceful lifting or pulling action, for example, pulling a plant out of the ground (Fig. 19.1), lifting a suitcase (Fig. 19.2), or falling on the shoulder, elbow, or hand (Fig. 19.3).

However, a specific injury or incident like one of these is not the most common cause of developing and prolonging shoulder pain. Overstretching or overloading the shoulder region due to positional stresses can be just as damaging. These stresses arise from prolonged or repeated raised arm activities performed while either standing or sitting, such as overhead building work (Fig. 19.4) or writing on a blackboard (Fig. 19.5).

Figure 19.2: . . . or lifting a suitcase . . .

Figure 19.3: . . . or in a fall onto the shoulder, elbow, or hand.

Figure 19.4: Overstretching or overloading the shoulder can occur in overhead work . . .

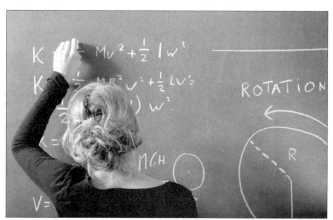

Figure 19.5: . . . or writing on a blackboard.

CONSEQUENCES OF POSTURAL NEGLECT

Unfortunately many of us spend much of our work and leisure time in a slouched position with the shoulders rounded or holding our arms in raised arm postures while performing activities. If you continue with these poor postures for long periods at a time and never regularly correct your slouched posture or take breaks from raised arm activities, you eventually lose the ability to bring the shoulders back into good alignment.

When these poor postures are maintained long enough, they cause overstretching or overloading of the structures in and around the shoulder. Thus, to begin with, pain will arise only in certain prolonged positions. However, once the poor postures become a habit and are maintained most of the time, movements of the arm as well as positions will produce pain. Shoulder problems developed in this way are the consequence of postural neglect. Poor shoulder and arm posture is not the only cause of shoulder pain. However, once shoulder problems have developed, poor posture will frequently make them worse and perpetuate them.

Some people who habitually adopt poor shoulder and arm postures, and remain unaware of the underlying cause, experience shoulder pain throughout their lifetime simply because they do not have the necessary information to correct the postural faults.

When pains of postural origin are first felt they are easily eliminated merely by correcting the postures. However, as time passes, these uncorrected habitual shoulder or raised arm postures cause changes to the structures of the shoulder. Excessive wear occurs, with loss of elasticity resulting in degenerative changes to the rotator cuff and other structures in and around the shoulder. The effects of poor posture in the long term, therefore, can be just as severe and harmful as the effects of injury.

The key things to learn are to:

- Sit and stand correctly.
- Interrupt any rounded neck and shoulder postures at regular intervals.

Try this simple test:

Sit in a slouched position with rounded shoulders (Fig. 19.6) and try to lift your arms above your head (Fig. 19.7). Hold for a few seconds and then lower them.

Next, sit up straight with upright posture (Fig. 19.8) and lift your arms again for a few seconds (Fig. 19.9).

Did you notice the difference? It is generally more difficult to lift the arms when you are slouched, as the shoulders are working at a mechanical disadvantage.

Figure 19.6: To learn how poor posture can cause injury, try sitting in a slouched position with rounded shoulders and . . .

Figure 19.7: . . . lifting your arms above your head.

Figure 19.8: Next, sit up straight with upright posture . . .

Figure 19.9: . . . and lift your arms again.

Now try the same test while standing. Stand in a slouched position with rounded shoulders (Fig. 19.10) and try to lift your arms above your head (Fig. 19.11). Hold for a few seconds and then lower them.

Figure 19.10: Try standing in a slouched position with rounded shoulders and . . .

Figure 19.11: . . . try to lift your arms above your head.

Figure 19.12: Next, stand up straight with upright posture and . . .

Figure 19.13: . . . lift your arms again.

Next, stand up straight with upright posture (Fig. 19.12) and lift your arms again for a few seconds (Fig. 19.13).

Again, did you notice the difference? More effort is required, you have a smaller range of motion, and the muscles fatigue more quickly in a slouched standing position. But these slouched postures are exactly the position from which we move our arms and shoulders much of the time without recognizing the role of poor posture in the onset and persistence of shoulder pain, as discussed above. Furthermore, particularly in our sedentary lifestyles, we seldom put our shoulders through a full range of motion. As a result they gradually lose their flexibility and the surrounding muscles lose their strength. These factors contribute to making us more prone to injury when we attempt a sudden lift or work with our arms above the level of our shoulders.

The main theme of this chapter is that pain of postural origin will not occur if you avoid prolonged overstretching or overloading of your shoulders. Should pain develop, there are certain movements or posture modifications you can perform in order to stop that pain. You should not have to seek assistance whenever posture-based pain arises.

POSTURAL STRESSES

The common postures and prolonged positions we adopt that affect the shoulder structures are primarily a combination of these three factors:

1. Performing repetitive or prolonged tasks with raised arm postures, such as welding or driving, and activities with our arms above shoulder height.
2. Sitting or standing in a slouched posture. The adverse effect of raised arm postures is increased if these activities are performed in slouched postural positions.
3. Lying and sleeping in positions that strain the shoulder.

Figure 19.14: Major factors contributing to shoulder pain are raised-arm or overhead activities such as gardening and . . .

Raised Arm Postures

Performing raised arm or overhead activities for prolonged periods of time (Figs. 19.14 and 19.15), or increasing the frequency or duration of such activities, is a major contributing factor to causing and perpetuating shoulder pain. Such activities place repeated or prolonged postural stresses on the structures of the shoulder.

Sitting and Standing for Long Periods

When we are moving about, especially when walking briskly and swinging the arms, we assume a fairly upright posture. The shoulder girdle is held directly over the vertebral column and consequently receives the maximum support possible. For most of us, however, sitting or standing for prolonged periods results in poor posture. When we stand for long periods (Fig. 19.16) or sit and relax in a chair (Fig. 19.17) for too

Figure 19.15: . . . working on a vehicle that is on a lift.

Figure 19.16: Poor posture can result from standing for long periods . . .

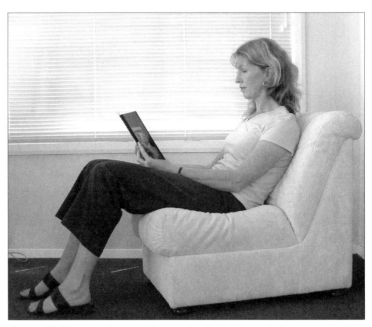

Figure 19.17: . . . or from sitting and relaxing in a chair.

long, the head slowly protrudes forward and the shoulder girdle becomes rounded because the supporting muscles become fatigued.

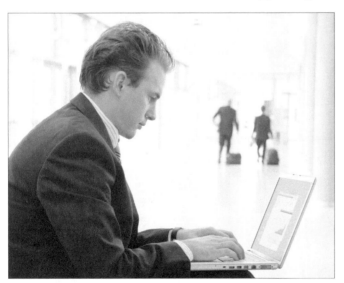

Figure 19.18: Slouched postures can be found in working in front of a computer, with outstretched arms.

As these muscles fatigue, they no longer hold us upright, and so we lose the main support for good shoulder posture. If we then perform raised arm activities from this poor posture, it further increases the load on the shoulder structures. Many of us spend increasing amounts of time at work or leisure in slouched postures, for example, in front of a computer (Fig. 19.18), with arms outstretched. Commonly our standing postures are just as harmful (Fig. 19.19).

Figure 19.19: Even upright postures, such as in welding, can be harmful.

Lying and Sleeping

If you wake up in the morning with a stiff and painful shoulder that was not causing problems the night before, or your shoulder pain wakes you consistently during the night, it is likely that something is wrong with the position you're sleeping in or with the support available for your shoulder.

If you lie in positions that place adverse stress on your shoulder, either by lying on it (Fig. 19.20), leaving it unsupported (Fig. 19.21), or leaving the arm raised (Fig. 19.22), a gradual overstretching or overloading of the painful structures occurs. Thus, poor sleeping postures can further an already painful shoulder.

ENVIRONMENTAL FACTORS

In order to successfully treat shoulder pain you must learn which arm or shoulder positions and activities aggravate and perpetuate your shoulder pain,

Figure 19.20: A gradual overstretching or overloading of the shoulder can occur when one lies on the shoulder, or . . .

Figure 19.22: . . . or lies in a raised-arm posture.

Figure 19.21: leaves it unsupported . . .

and what are the correct positions and ways to perform activities that will enable you to relieve your pain and regain your function. As discussed, it is occupations or activities that have one's arms raised in static positions, or performing repetitive overhead activities, that gradually result in overloading, overstretching, or compressing of the shoulder structures (Figs. 19.23–25).

These so-called gradual process or overuse conditions often begin as a minor irritation felt in the shoulder region. This is at first eased temporarily by changing the position of the arm or shoulder and therefore is often ignored. However, if you continue to apply these overloading activities, the

Figure 19.23: Having the arms raised in a static position, or in performing repetitive overhead activities, gradually results in overloading, overstretching, or compressing of the shoulder structures.

Figure 19.24: Another example of how having the arms raised can cause problems

affected structures have no chance to recover and they gradually weaken to the point that even minor strains cause pain. When this occurs your condition becomes long-standing, and pain becomes persistent. There are several factors that result in, or aggravate, shoulder pain that you need to learn to recognize:

- Increasing the time you spend in an occupation with raised arm or repetitive work actions.
- Undertaking an activity that is either new to you or one that you have not performed for a period of time. If you introduce new stresses on

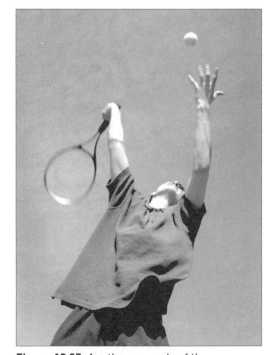

Figure 19.25: Another example of the same

the shoulder, such as an increased load, too rapidly, the structures of the shoulder cannot adapt.

- Performing activities that have you holding your arms in raised positions for prolonged periods or performing repeated movements away from your body or above shoulder height. Sustaining these positions places a harmful load on the structures of the shoulder.

- Using inappropriate equipment, for example, attempting to trim a hedge with blunt shears.

- Working in a confined or restricted space, forcing you to adopt inappropriate or uncomfortable positions of your arms and shoulders in order to perform the tasks.

Over a period of hours, days, or weeks, one or several of these factors can have a cumulative effect on the structures of your shoulder, resulting in shoulder pain developing.

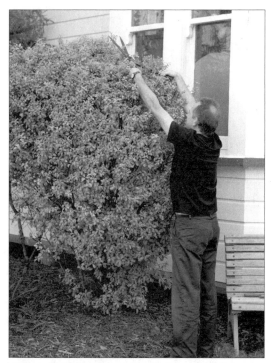

Figure 19.26: Incorrect position, making the person vulnerable to shoulder pain or injury

HOW TO MANAGE PROLONGED OR REPEATED USE OF RAISED ARM POSITIONS

It is necessary to avoid or limit activities that have our arms raised in front, to the side, or above our shoulder or head, because these place the structures of the shoulder in their weakest position and make them most vulnerable to becoming painful or injured (Figs. 19.26, 19.28, and 19.30). Always adopt a position where your arms or elbows are close to your body—either by your sides or just in front of you (Figs. 19.27 and 19.29)—and if you're performing a heavy task, such as drilling, use both arms (Fig. 19.31); this is the position of strength and stability for the structures of the shoulder and it will reduce, minimize, or prevent the onset of shoulder pain.

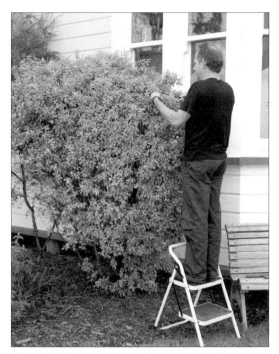

Figure 19.27: Correct position, making the person less vulnerable

Figure 19.28: Incorrect position, making the person vulnerable

Figure 19.29: Correct position, making the person less vulnerable

If you are unable to avoid prolonged raised arm activities, or are about to commence a raised arm activity that you do infrequently, perform the activity for only a short period of time. Then stop the activity just as you are feeling some discomfort in your shoulder region and pause for thirty seconds or so. This will allow the structures of your shoulder to recover, and it'll enable you to develop the habit of appropriately pacing your activities.

You can also use this time to perform this simple stretch:

Stand upright (Fig. 19.32), clasp your hands behind your back (Fig. 19.33), and pull your shoulders and arms backward as if trying to pull the shoulder blades together (Fig. 19.34). Hold for three seconds and repeat three to five times.

Figure 19.30: Incorrect position, making the person vulnerable

Figure 19.31: Correct position, making the person less vulnerable

Figure 19.32: To perform a simple stretch, stand upright . . .

Figure 19.33: . . . clasp your hands behind your back . . .

Figure 19.34: . . . and pull your shoulders and arms backward as if trying to pull the shoulder blades together.

Regularly varying your daily tasks, or taking a thirty-second break every ten minutes from these potentially harmful activities, will minimize the chances of developing or aggravating a shoulder problem.

Some tasks can be performed only in positions that are likely to cause over-stretching or overloading of the shoulders. They may have to be performed in cramped spaces or with head and shoulder in awkward static positions, particularly if the arms are above the level of the shoulders (Fig. 19.35).

Figure 19.35: Some tasks can be performed only in positions likely to cause overstretching or overloading of the shoulder.

Under these circumstances you may not be able to prevent the onset of shoulder pain by one measure alone, whether regularly assuming the correct arm posture, taking regular rests, or performing a pain-relieving exercise. If your shoulder problems are brought on in this way you must frequently interrupt these adverse postures by taking a thirty-second break every few minutes and perform the stretch described above. It is also necessary to perform this type of task for only a limited time and then either take a prolonged rest or change activity to avoid injury to your shoulder.

HOW TO MANAGE PROLONGED SITTING OR STANDING

You may have been sitting slouched for many years without shoulder pain. However, once you have developed shoulder problems you must no longer sit in the old way, because this posture will only continue overloading the shoulder structures. Very commonly, while sitting, you will have insufficient support for your lower back, neck, and shoulders, and you will continue to stress these areas when you are at a computer, reading, or relaxing. If your shoulder problems are aggravated by reading, computer use, or watching television, the posture that you have adopted is the cause of the pain, and this posture depends to a large extent on the type of chair or support you use.

During sitting, the position of the lower back strongly influences the posture of the neck and shoulder area. Therefore it is necessary to first correct the posture of your lower back. How to assume and maintain the correct posture of the lower back when sitting is described fully in Chapter 4. However, for the purposes of this chapter, you must be fully aware of the following:

If the lower back is allowed to slouch, it is impossible to sit with head and shoulders pulled back as they should be (Fig. 19.36). To sit correctly, you must maintain the natural hollow (lordosis) that is present in your lower back while standing (Fig. 19.37). To maintain your lordosis it is helpful to use a lumbar roll; this is a specially designed support for your lower back (Fig. 19.38). Without this support your lower back slouches, your head protrudes, and your

Figure 19.36: If the lower back is allowed to slouch, it is impossible to sit with the head and shoulders pulled backward.

Figure 19.37: To sit correctly, you must maintain the natural hollow (lordosis) that is present in your lower back when you are standing.

shoulders become rounded as soon as you relax or concentrate on anything other than your posture. To counteract this slouching, place a lumbar roll in the small of your back, about waist level, whenever you are sitting. See Appendix B for information on where to purchase a lumbar roll and other spinal support products.

Figure 19.38: To maintain your lordosis, it is helpful to use a lumbar roll that is specially designed to support your lower back.

When first using these procedures to correct your lower back, neck, and shoulder posture in sitting, you will experience some new pains. These may be different from your original pain and may be felt in another place. New pains are the result of performing new exercises and maintaining new positions. They should be expected and will wear off in a few days, provided postural correction is continued on a regular basis. Once you have become used to sitting correctly, you will enjoy it. You will soon notice the reduction or absence of pain and the increased comfort. From then on you will automatically choose chairs that allow you to sit more correctly.

Sales of the Original McKenzie range of spinal supports provide funding for research into improved methods of treatment for musculoskeletal disorders and to provide relevant education for both health care professionals and patients. These spinal supports are available worldwide from distributors listed on the Spinal Publications NZ Ltd website (www.spinalpublications.co.nz). Also see Appendix B, "Products for the Back and Neck."

Correcting the standing posture is similar to correcting the sitting posture in that generally we need to move from a slouched position to a more upright stance (Fig. 19.32). However, as well as standing erect you may also clasp your hands behind your back, as described earlier (Fig. 19.33), and pull your shoulders backward as if trying to pull the shoulder blades together (Fig. 19.34). Sustain this position for a few seconds and repeat three or four times. This can also be performed while you are walking.

Figure 19.39: Try using an additional pillow or a more supportive one.

Figure 19.40: Try sleeping on your back with a pillow under your shoulder.

HOW TO MANAGE LYING AND SLEEPING

There are two things to consider with shoulder pain that arises from lying or sleeping.

If you lie on your painful shoulder this will place a compressive load on the area and often can be tolerated for only a short period of time before you have to change position. The best solution for postural pain that disturbs your sleep when lying on the painful side is to train yourself not to lie on that side for any length of time. Another common solution is to take some of the load off the painful shoulder by correcting the sleeping surface. Try using a larger pillow, or an additional, more supportive one, that you can adjust to maintain normal alignment of the neck (Fig. 19.39). If this does not provide relief it is recommended you either sleep on your back, with a pillow under your shoulder to provide support (Fig. 19.40), or sleep on your nonpainful side as discussed.

THE KEYS TO PREVENTION

Remember these practices to prevent the development or recurrence of shoulder pain:

- Adjust your environment and posture to enable you to have your arms in the correct position with elbows close to your body for as much of the time as possible.

- Interrupt sustained raised arm positions with frequent rests and stretching.
- Vary or rotate tasks at regular intervals to prevent putting a prolonged load on specific structures.
- Learn to sit and stand upright, and to lie and sleep with the neck and shoulder region well supported.

FROZEN SHOULDER

One relatively common and frustrating source of shoulder pain is called a "frozen shoulder" or capsulitis. This is a condition where movement of the shoulder in all directions becomes both painful and increasingly stiff (Figs. 19.41–44).

The condition frequently affects people over the age of forty and may

Figure 19.41: A painful position in "frozen shoulder"

Figure 19.42: Another one

Figure 19.43: A third one

Figure 19.44: And finally a fourth

come on for no apparent reason, though it sometimes develops following an injury to the shoulder, wrist, or hand, such as a severe sprain or fracture. Middle-aged women and diabetics seem to have a higher incidence of this condition, although the reasons for this are unclear.

A frozen shoulder is frequently described as going through three stages:

1. The first stage is when the shoulder becomes increasingly more painful during the day and begins to disturb sleep, but remains reasonably mobile.

2. The second stage sees the shoulder become increasingly stiff and painful, often severely restricting the performance of activities at work and daily life, and disturbing sleep. Attempting to exercise the arm to prevent this stiffness occurring may be very painful.

3. The third stage sees the shoulder gradually become less and less painful but remain stiff until gradually it regains most, or all, of its previously lost mobility. Exercises are frequently successful during this stage in promoting the restoration of movement in the shoulder.

Each stage may take three months or longer and the whole process from onset to resolution of the condition may take a frustrating twelve to eighteen months or longer.

Chapter 22 will explain how to determine if your frozen shoulder will benefit from the treatment described in this book.

The information regarding posture is still an important component in minimizing your shoulder pain during this process.

20 THE MCKENZIE METHOD FOR THE SHOULDER

THE AIM OF THE EXERCISES

The purpose of the shoulder exercises is to stop pain and, where possible, restore normal function; that is, to regain full mobility in the shoulder or as much movement as possible under the given circumstances.

When you are exercising for pain relief, you should move to the edge of the pain or just into the pain, then release the pressure and return to the starting position. As you release the stretch, the pain must diminish back to the starting level or less. If it does not, you are overdoing it. Use less force. When you are exercising for stiffness, the exercises can be made more effective by firmly and steadily applying overpressure (as described in Chapter 12) in order to obtain the maximum amount of movement. Postural correction and maintenance of the correct posture should always occur during and following the exercises. Once you no longer have shoulder pain, ongoing good postural habits are essential to prevent the recurrence of shoulder problems.

Your understanding of this chapter is essential for successful self-treatment. Please read it carefully.

Effect on Pain Intensity and Location

You can look for three main effects while performing the exercises:

1. They may cause the symptoms to disappear.
2. They may cause an increase or decrease in the intensity of the pain that you experience.
3. They may cause the pain to move from where you usually feel it to some other location.

The effects of the exercises on the intensity or location of the pain can sometimes be very rapid. It is possible that completing as few as ten or fifteen movements will reduce the intensity or change the location of the pain, and in some conditions the pain can completely disappear. However, in other cases this improvement may be noticed over several days or up to a few weeks.

In order to determine whether the exercise program is good for you, it is very important that you observe closely any changes in the location of the pain. You may notice that, as a result of the exercises, pain originally felt on the outside of the upper arm, or down the arm, moves toward the point of your shoulder. In other words, your pain may become more localized in the shoulder.

PAIN INTENSITY

If your shoulder pain is of such intensity that you can move your arm only with difficulty and cannot find a position to lie comfortably in bed, your approach to the exercises should be cautious and unhurried.

On commencing any of the exercises you may experience an initial increase in pain. This is common and can be expected. As you continue to practice, the pain should quickly diminish, at least to its former level. Usually this occurs during the first exercise session. This will often be followed by the pain becoming less strong in the arm and more localized to the shoulder joint. Once the pain no longer spreads down the arm and is felt in the shoulder only, the intensity of the pain will steadily decrease over a period of a few days. When you continue the exercises, the pain will often disappear entirely.

If, following an initial pain increase, the pain continues to increase in intensity or spreads to places farther away from the shoulder, such as farther down the arm or up to the neck, you should stop exercising and seek advice from a McKenzie-trained practitioner. In other words, do not continue with any of the exercises if your symptoms are much worse immediately after exercising and remain worse the next day. Also discontinue if, as you exercise, symptoms arise or intensify in the arm below the elbow.

As noted, once you have started this exercise program, you should expect new pains to develop. These are different from your original pain and are usually felt in parts of the shoulder area that were previously not affected. New pains are the result of performing movements your body is not used to and, provided you continue with the exercises, the pains will wear off in three to four days.

If your symptoms have been present rather continuously for many weeks or months, you should not expect to be pain free in two to three days. The response may be slower, but, if you are doing the correct exercises, it will only be a matter of time before the pain subsides.

As long as your pain is slowly improving, continue with the exercises that have led to this improvement. Do not change anything in your established routine. It may be tempting to add other exercises, but this may disrupt your progress. Wait until improvement stops before considering any other activity or exercise.

STARTING THE EXERCISE PROGRAM

When you commence this exercise program you should stop any other exercises that you may have been shown elsewhere or happen to do regularly—for example, for fitness or sport. If you want to continue with exercises other than the ones described in this book for shoulder problems, you should wait until your pain has subsided completely. As long as your pain is slowly improving, continue with the exercises that have led to this improvement. Do not change anything in your established routine. It may be tempting to add other exercises, but this may disrupt your progress. Wait until improvement stops before considering any other activity or exercise.

We recommend that you adopt the standing position when learning to perform the exercises.

21 THE MCKENZIE METHOD EXERCISES FOR THE SHOULDER

OVERVIEW

In the preceding chapters we outlined the conditions that can cause pain, reduce mobility, and limit function in your shoulder. As discussed in Chapter 17, it is sometimes difficult to determine exactly what shoulder condition you have.

Therefore it is vital to follow the exercise sequence exactly as outlined in Chapters 21 and 22, as it is a systematic approach that will enable you to successfully treat your own shoulder condition.

The exercises are described and clearly illustrated in this chapter, while Chapter 22 details more information as to when to apply the exercises and the responses that may be expected. We recommend that you try each of the exercises described below with your pain-free arm first, and then cautiously attempt the same exercise with your painful arm. In this way you can compare the pain and range of motion in both arms. By commencing the exercise program as described in Chapter 22, you can attempt to improve the painful arm until it feels and moves the same way as your pain-free arm.

It is strongly recommended that you familiarize yourself with the exercises and information in Chapters 21 and 22 before commencing the program.

SHOULDER EXERCISE 1

Shoulder Pendular Exercise

A pendular exercise is a slow swinging of the arm in a pain-free arc of motion, like the pendulum in a grandfather clock.

This exercise is used mainly in the treatment of significant shoulder pain, and it can be useful in reducing the pain brought on during the night or in the morning by sleeping on your painful side, or the sudden pain you may get when placing your painful arm into a sleeve while dressing.

Stand up and then position yourself leaning forward, supporting yourself with your good arm on a table or chair, with your painful shoulder hanging down. Allow your painful shoulder to relax completely (Fig. 21.1). Now you are ready to start the first exercise.

Slowly swing your arm backward and forward in an arc of motion that is pain free (Figs. 21.2–4). As with the back and neck exercises, you will use the right amount of time with each use of each exercise if you say to yourself, "pressure on, pressure off."

Figure 21.1: Allow your painful shoulder to relax completely. Now you are ready to start Exercise 1.

If this movement is painful, perform the exercise in a smaller arc of motion so the movement is pain free. Some people find that holding a small weight—such as a can of food or a small dumbbell—in the hand while performing this exercise also assists in reducing pain.

When used in the treatment of shoulder pain the exercise should be repeated ten times per session, with the sessions spread evenly six to eight times throughout the day until you go to bed at night. This means you should repeat the sessions about every two hours.

Figure 21.2: Slowly swing your arm backward and forward in an arc of motion that is pain free.

Figure 21.3: A second illustration of this exercise motion

Figure 21.4: A third illustration of the same

SHOULDER EXERCISE 2

Shoulder Extension in Standing

Extension here means reaching your arm backward. This exercise can be used in both the treatment and the prevention of shoulder pain, and it is particularly useful if you have more pain or less movement than in your pain-free shoulder when you attempt this exercise.

Stand upright with your head and shoulders pulled back (Fig. 21.5). Now you are ready to start Shoulder Exercise 2.

Reach the straight arm of your painful shoulder behind your back (Fig. 21.6). Now with your pain-free arm slowly push the painful arm farther away from your back until you feel a firm stretch at your painful shoulder (Figs. 21.7 and 21.8).

Figure 21.5: Stand upright with your head and shoulders pulled back. Now you are ready for Exercise 2.

Figure 21.6: Place the arm of the painful shoulder behind your back.

Figure 21.7: With your pain-free arm, slowly push the painful arm away from your back until you feel a firm stretch in your painful shoulder.

Figure 21.8: This is a different illustration of the motion in Figure 21.7.

Once you have held this position for a few seconds, you should return your arm to the starting position. Each time you perform this movement cycle, try to push your arm backward a little farther so that in the end you have reached the maximum possible degree of extension.

When you have reached the stage where you are comfortable pushing your arm behind you as far as possible with your pain-free arm, increase the effect

Figure 21.9: When you are comfortable pushing your arm behind you as far as possible, take the exercise a step further by using your pain-free arm and holding a pole, golf club, or broomstick in both hands.

of the exercise by using a pole, golf club, or broomstick to gain more leverage and reach (Fig. 21.9).

Another method of taking the arm to the end of its range is to place your hand, palm down, on a waist-high surface such as a chair, sideboard, or window frame (Fig. 21.10). Then slowly bend your knees to apply overpressure to the extension exercise (Fig. 21.11). The higher you place your arm, the less you will have to bend your knees to produce an effective stretch.

When this exercise is used in the treatment of shoulder pain, Shoulder Exercise 2 should be repeated ten times per session and the sessions should be spread evenly six to eight times throughout the day until you go to bed at night. This means you should repeat the sessions about every two hours.

Figure 21.10: Place your hand "palm-down" on a surface such as a chair, sideboard, or window frame.

Figure 21.11: Then slowly bend your knees to apply overpressure to the exercise you are doing.

SHOULDER EXERCISE 3

Shoulder Internal Rotation in Standing

Internal rotation means placing your hand up behind your back. This exercise can be used in both the treatment and the prevention of shoulder pain, and it is particularly useful if you have more pain or less movement than in your pain-free shoulder when you attempt this exercise.

Stand upright with your head and shoulders pulled back (Fig. 21.12).

Figure 21.12: Stand upright with your head and shoulders pulled back.

Figure 21.13: Place the arm of your painful shoulder behind your back.

Figure 21.14: Now, with your pain-free arm, slowly push the painful arm up your back until you feel a firm stretch in your painful shoulder.

Figure 21.15: Another illustration of the previous action but with the painful arm raised higher

Place the arm of your painful shoulder behind your back (Fig. 21.13). Now, with your pain-free arm, slowly push the painful arm up your back until you feel a firm stretch in your painful shoulder (Figs. 21.14 and 21.15).

Figure 21.16: To take the exercise further, use a towel.

Figure 21.17: Still using a towel, use your pain-free arm to pull the arm of your painful shoulder up your back.

Once you have held this position for a few seconds, you should return your arm to the starting position. Each time you perform this movement cycle, try to push your arm up your back a little farther so that in the end you have reached the maximum possible internal rotation.

When you have reached the stage where you are comfortable pushing your arm up your back, increase the effect of the exercise by using a towel for increased leverage (Fig. 21.16) and pull the arm of your painful shoulder up your back with your pain-free arm (Fig. 21.17).

When used in the treatment of shoulder pain, Shoulder Exercise 3 should be repeated ten times per session and the sessions should be spread evenly six to eight times throughout the day until you go to bed at night. This means you should repeat the sessions about every two hours. If this is very painful, start with four repetitions, four to six times a day, and increase as you are able to do so.

If your pain is too severe to tolerate Shoulder Exercise 3, you should discontinue it and go back to performing Shoulder Exercise 2 for a few more days, before trying it again.

SHOULDER EXERCISE 4

Shoulder Elevation in Lying

Elevation means lifting your arms forward and upward. This exercise can be used if you have pain or difficulty in attempting to lift your arm in front of you in standing. It is a way of gradually improving this movement before commencing Shoulder Exercise 5, Shoulder Elevation in Standing.

Lie faceup on a bed or the floor. Rest your head and shoulders flat; do not use a pillow (Fig. 21.18). Now you are ready to start Shoulder Exercise 4.

Interlock the fingers of both hands. Slowly raise your arms over your head (Fig. 21.19), using the pain-free arm to assist the arm of the painful or stiff shoulder until you feel a firm stretch in your affected shoulder.

Once you have held this position for a few seconds, you should return your arm to the starting position. Each time you perform this movement cycle try to push your arms back a little farther so that in the end you have reached the maximum possible reach (Fig. 21.20).

When used in the treatment of shoulder pain or stiffness, Shoulder Exercise 4 should be repeated ten times per session and the sessions should be spread evenly six to eight times throughout the day until you go to bed at night. This means you should repeat the sessions about every two hours.

Figure 21.18: Lie faceup on a bed or the floor. Rest your head and shoulders flat; do not use a pillow. Now you are ready for Exercise 4.

Figure 21.19: Interlock the fingers of both hands. Slowly raise your arms straight up and then back, over your head.

SHOULDER EXERCISE 5

Shoulder Elevation in Standing

Figure 21.20: Return your arms to the starting position, but each time you repeat the cycle of movements, try to extend your arms a little farther so that at the end you have reached the maximum possible distance from your head.

Elevation means lifting your arms forward and upward.

Stand upright with your head and shoulders pulled back. Take a cloth in the hand of your painful or stiff shoulder and hold it against a smooth wall or door frame (Fig. 21.21). Now slowly slide your hand up the wall until you feel a firm stretch in your painful or stiff shoulder (Fig. 21.22).

Once you have held this position for a few seconds, you should return your arm to the starting position (Fig. 21.23). Each time you perform this movement cycle try to push your arm up a little farther so that in the end you have reached the maximum possible elevation (Fig. 21.22).

When used in the treatment of shoulder pain or stiffness, Shoulder Exercise 5 should be repeated ten times per session and the sessions should be spread evenly six to eight times throughout the day until you go to bed at

Figure 21.21: Stand upright with your head and shoulders pulled back and hold a cloth in the hand of your painful or stiff shoulder against a wall or door frame.

Figure 21.22: Now slowly slide your hand and cloth up the wall until you feel a firm stretch in your painful or stiff shoulder.

Figure 21.23: Same photo as with Figure 21.21. Once you have held the above position for a few seconds, return your arm to the starting position.

night. If you do the exercise eight times a day, this means you should repeat the sessions about every two hours.

If your pain is too severe to tolerate Exercise 5, you should discontinue it and go back to performing Exercise 4 for a few more days, before trying Exercise 5 again.

SHOULDER EXERCISE 6

Shoulder Strengthening— Isometric Abduction in Standing

Isometric means static tensioning, and *abduction* means pushing your arm sideways, away from the body. This exercise is a way to begin to strengthen the rotator cuff muscles and tendons around the shoulder once your range of motion has recovered but you still have some pain. Instructions on when to apply this exercise are further described in Chapter 22.

Stand upright with your painful side near a wall. Make sure your feet are apart and your arm is relaxed by your side (Fig. 21.24). Slowly push the outside of the hand of your painful arm against the wall until you feel a firm tension in your shoulder—but do not allow further movement of your arm or body (Fig. 21.25). Hold this position for a few seconds, then return your arm to the starting position. Each time you perform this movement cycle, try to apply more pressure against the wall so that in the end you are able to place a firm tension with some discomfort during each repetition of the exercise. However, any discomfort that is produced must disappear within a few minutes of completing each set of ten repetitions.

When used in the treatment of shoulder pain, Shoulder Exercise 6 should be repeated ten times per session and the sessions should be spread evenly six to eight times throughout the day until you go to bed at night. If you do the exercise eight times, this means you should repeat the sessions about every two hours.

Figure 21.24: Stand upright with your painful side near a wall. Make sure your feet are apart and your painful arm is relaxed by your side.

Figure 21.25: Slowly push the outside of the hand of your painful arm against the wall until you feel a firm tension in your shoulder—but do not allow further movement of your arm or the rest of your body.

22 WHEN TO DO THE SHOULDER EXERCISES

> You should seek advice from your doctor if your shoulder pain is of such severity that it is impossible to perform these exercises (or other exercises in this book) or your pain is becoming intolerable.

Figure 22.1: Shoulder Pendular Exercise. For details, please see Exercise 1 in the introduction to Chapter 21.

WHEN YOU ARE IN SIGNIFICANT PAIN

If the pain is severe you will find certain movements impossible to do, and it may be difficult to perform your daily activities or find a comfortable position in which to rest. Even though you have significant pain, you should always attempt to commence with Shoulder Exercise 1, Shoulder Pendular Exercise (Fig. 22.1).

Many people find this exercise gives substantial relief from pain. It is also very important to follow the postural education in Chapter

19 in an attempt to find resting positions where you are as comfortable as possible when sitting, standing, and lying.

When you have reached the stage, over the next two days to two weeks, where either your pain decreases or you are able to start to move your arm behind your back, you can progress to Shoulder Exercise 2, Shoulder Extension in Standing (Figs. 22.2–5).

Figure 22.2: Exercise 2, Shoulder Extension in Standing

Figure 22.3: Progress in Exercise 2

Figure 22.4: Further movement in this exercise

Figure 22.5: End of this exercise

You should seek advice from your doctor if your shoulder pain is of such severity that you find it impossible to perform this exercise or your pain is becoming intolerable.

WHEN ACUTE PAIN HAS SUBSIDED

When acute or severe pain has subsided, or you have only intermittent pain, you may still feel some pain when moving your arm in certain ways. Commonly, you will notice this when raising your arm out to the side or attempting

Figure 22.6: Start with the last part of Exercise 2.

to reach behind your back. It is likely that at this stage of your shoulder condition, healing of the overstretched or damaged soft tissues has taken place.

Now you must ensure that the elasticity, strength, and flexibility of your shoulder are restored without causing further damage. This is the aim of the structured exercise sequence outlined in this chapter.

Nevertheless, in a few cases you will find, by performing Shoulder Exercises 2 to 5, that the range of motion in your painful arm matches that in your pain-free arm and you can perform all these exercises with no discomfort. If this applies to you, you may move directly to Shoulder Exercise 6 in order to strengthen your shoulder.

To Start the Recovery

Begin with Shoulder Exercise 2, Shoulder Extension in Standing (Fig. 22.6). Repeat the exercise up to ten times. Each time you repeat the exercise you must move to the edge of the pain and then release the pressure. Over a few days you will generally find that the movement begins to improve,

Figure 22.7: Using a broomstick or pole, you can progress in this exercise.

Figure 22.8: Or a chair

Figure 22.9: Shoulder Rotation in Standing

Figure 22.10: Progress in the same exercise

Figure 22.11: Further progress in this exercise

and you can increase the effect of this exercise to ensure you are getting to the end of your range of motion by using the pole or furniture as described in Chapter 21 (Figs. 22.7 and 22.8).

Each time you repeat the exercise you must move to the edge of the pain and then release the pressure. It may take several days or up to a few weeks before you are able to progress to the next exercise, but as soon as you can perform Exercise 2 comfortably, progress to Shoulder Exercise 3, Shoulder Internal Rotation in Standing (Figs. 22.9–11).

Repeat Exercise 3 up to ten times. Each time you repeat the exercise you must move to the edge of the pain and then release the pressure. Your pain should decrease and disappear entirely over a period of several days, or up to a few weeks, as this movement improves. You should be able to take your affected arm up your back as comfortably as you can take your pain-free arm, and you should be able to progress to using a towel to ensure you are getting to the end of your range of motion (Fig. 22.12).

Once you are able to perform Exercise 3 comfortably with a towel

Figure 22.12: You can use a towel to ensure you are getting to the end of your range.

and have obtained the same range of motion as you have in your pain-free arm, you will generally have noticed a significant decrease in your shoulder pain. In many cases the pain will have stopped, and you will also have noticed an increase in the functional use of your arm during your daily activities. If this is the case, you are well on your way to recovering the strength in your shoulder muscles as you gradually increase your activities. Even so, do not forget the important postural education in Chapter 19 to prevent the onset of your pain at rest. Once you are completely symptom free and have no pain or stiffness, follow the guidelines in that chapter to prevent recurrence of shoulder problems.

If you have practiced Shoulder Exercises 2 and 3 for two weeks without noticing any improvement in your ability to raise your arm in front of you, you can begin Shoulder Exercise 4, Shoulder Elevation in Lying (Fig. 22.13).

Figure 22.13: The beginning of Exercise 4, Shoulder Elevation in Lying

Figure 22.14: Once you can perform Exercise 4 comfortably, you can move to Exercise 5, Shoulder Elevation in Standing.

Repeat the exercise up to ten times. Each time you repeat the motion you must move to the edge of the pain and then release the pressure. That is, you must feel some discomfort during each repetition of the exercise. However, any discomfort following the set of exercises must settle within a few minutes. In some cases it may take a few weeks to restore the ability to reach above your head. Still, as soon as you are able to perform this exercise comfortably, you can progress to Shoulder Exercise 5, Shoulder Elevation in Standing (Fig. 22.14).

Repeat the exercise up to ten times, following the instructions above. Again it may take several days to a few weeks before you are able to take your affected arm above your head with comfort. If Exercise 5 is painful to perform, continue with Exercise 4 for a few weeks before attempting it again.

If you feel only stiffness on these movements, rather than pain, you should do the same exercises but apply more overpressure at the end of each movement. By exercising in this way you achieve movement to the maximum possible degree. In most cases you should have restored normal function within three to six weeks.

When you have restored the normal range of motion to your affected shoulder and are able to perform Shoulder Exercises 2, 3, 4, and 5 fully with no pain, you will most likely find that you no longer have shoulder pain and have regained the functional use of your affected shoulder.

Once you are completely symptom free and have no pain or stiffness, you should follow the guidelines in Chapter 19 to prevent recurrence of shoulder problems.

If you have carefully followed the exercise sequence for a few weeks, and you have not achieved the ability to perform Exercises 2, 3, 4, and 5 comfortably, refer to the section below, "When You Have a Frozen Shoulder," for treatment guidelines.

WHEN YOU GET NO RESPONSE OR BENEFIT

When you continue to experience shoulder pain in raised arm activities, yet are able to perform Exercises 2, 3, 4, and 5, you may need to strengthen the rotator cuff muscles and tendons around your shoulder. If this is the case, you should begin doing Shoulder Exercise 6, Shoulder Strengthening—Isometric Abduction in Standing (Fig. 22.15).

Repeat the exercise up to ten times. Each time you repeat the motion you must move to the edge of the pain and then release the pressure. However, any discomfort that is produced must settle within a few minutes of completing each set of ten repetitions.

By exercising this way you place the appropriate loading on the shoulder area required to stimulate a recovery in the affected structures around your shoulder.

Figure 22.15: Exercise 6, Shoulder Strengthening— Isometric Abduction

In most cases you will notice the pain gradually decreasing over a three-week period, and by six to twelve weeks you should have a largely pain-free shoulder.

WHEN YOU HAVE NO PAIN OR STIFFNESS

Many people with shoulder problems have lengthy spells in which they experience little or no pain. If you have had one or more episodes of shoulder pain, you should start the exercise program even though you may be pain free at the moment. In this situation, however, it is not necessary to do all the exercises or to exercise every two hours.

To prevent recurrence of shoulder problems you should perform Shoulder Exercise 3, Shoulder Internal Rotation in Standing (Fig. 22.16), followed by Exercise 5, Shoulder Elevation in Standing (Fig. 22.17), a couple of times a day to ensure you maintain the shoulder's range of motion.

Figure 22.16: Exercise 3, Shoulder Internal Rotation in Standing

Figure 22.17: Exercise 5, Shoulder Elevation in Standing

Figure 22.18: Exercise 6, Shoulder Strengthening— Isometric Abduction

If Exercise 6, Shoulder Strengthening—Isometric Abduction in Standing (Fig. 22.18), has been the exercise sequence that has relieved your shoulder symptoms, perform this exercise instead.

Perform these exercises on a regular basis, preferably in the morning and at night. Furthermore, whenever you feel pain developing, whether it's during activity or work or while sitting and relaxing, you should perform them. As it takes only a few minutes to perform one session of these exercises, lack of time should never be used as an excuse for not doing them.

It is even more important that you watch your shoulder posture at all times and never again let postural stresses be the cause of shoulder pain. The exercises described in this book will have very little or no effect if you constantly fall back into your previous poor shoulder postures and raised arm positions. While it may be necessary to exercise in the manner described above for the rest of your life, it is absolutely essential that you develop and maintain good postural habits.

A graduated increase in activities that generally improve your fitness should also be considered. Even a regular walking program will assist in maintaining upright posture and arm mobility, while appropriately structured gym programs, aerobic activities, or fitness classes will specifically assist with flexibility and strength in the neck and shoulder girdle.

Yoga, tai chi, and martial arts are activities that specifically promote postural awareness while also using exercises that will ensure the shoulders and arms are put through a wide range of motion.

WHEN YOU HAVE A FROZEN SHOULDER

As described in Chapter 19, a frozen shoulder goes through three stages. In stage one the shoulder becomes increasingly painful but remains mobile. During the second stage the shoulder becomes increasingly less mobile in all directions while remaining painful. To assess the state of your shoulder we recommend you perform Shoulder Exercises 1, 2, and 3 for three weeks— initially very cautiously if required by your pain response. If there is no improvement in your pain and no increase in your shoulder movement in any direction, we recommend that you see a physician to confirm your condition.

He or she may be able to offer you some benefit from a course of medication or refer you for some other intervention as appropriate.

In the third state of a frozen shoulder, when your shoulder becomes less painful but remains stiff, we recommend you continue with the exercise program for three to six months. An increase in range of motion and functional movement with everyday tasks can be very slow but in most cases the result eventually is a very good recovery.

The exercises described in this book will have very little or no effect if you constantly fall back into your previous poor shoulder postures and raised arm positions.

WHEN YOU HAVE A RECURRENCE

At the first sign of recurrence of shoulder pain, you should immediately perform the exercises that have previously helped you.

If your pain is already too severe to tolerate these exercises or if they fail to reduce the pain, you must quickly introduce Shoulder Exercise 1, Shoulder Pendular Exercise, and Exercise 2, Shoulder Extension in Standing, and then gradually work through the exercise sequence. Again, you must pay extra attention to your shoulder posture, regularly perform postural correction, and maintain the correct posture as much as you can when sitting, standing, and lying.

If you continue to have shoulder pain and a loss of function, we recommend you seek advice from a health professional, ideally a credentialed member or associate of the McKenzie Institute. To obtain the names of these practitioners in your area, see Appendix A.

APPENDIX A

HOW TO FIND A MCKENZIE-TRAINED HEALTH CARE PRACTITIONER

TO LOCATE A PHYSICAL THERAPIST, CHIROPRACTOR, OR PHYSICIAN WHO is a credentialed member or associate of the McKenzie Institute International, telephone the institute's U.S. branch at (800) 635-8380 or its Canadian branch at (800) 463-8568. You may also visit the McKenzie Institute's website at www.mckenziemdt.org.

Members of the McKenzie Institute worldwide are available to appear at schools to provide group education and instruction to schoolchildren in the correction of posture. The institute has an educational video to assist in this program. There is no charge for either an appearance by a member of the institute or the video. For further information, contact a credentialed member or associate of the McKenzie Institute.

THE MCKENZIE INSTITUTE INTERNATIONAL

The McKenzie Institute International main website, www.mckenziemdt.org, includes information about:

- Robin McKenzie
- The McKenzie Method of Mechanical Diagnosis and Therapy
- The McKenzie Institute International
- The McKenzie Institute's education programs

The website can also help you find:

- Certified McKenzie clinics
- Clinicians holding a McKenzie Institute diploma or credentialing certificate
- Your local branch

> The McKenzie Institute International Head Office
> 3 Alexander Road, P.O. Box 2026
> Raumati Beach 5255, New Zealand
> Website: www.mckenziemdt.org
> E-mail: mckinst@xtra.co.nz
> Phone: +64 4 299-6645
> Fax: +64 4 299-7010

There are now twenty-six McKenzie Institute branches serving thirty-two countries, up from twenty-one serving twenty-three in the original edition of this book, published in 2000. Here are all the countries with branches or (in six cases) a "branch presence" served by a branch in another country: Argentina, Australia, Austria (served by Germany), Belgium (served by Netherlands), Brazil, Canada, Croatia, Cyprus (served by Greece), Czech Republic, Denmark, Finland, France, Germany, Greece, Hungary, India, Ireland (served by United Kingdom), Italy, Japan, Luxembourg (served by Netherlands), Netherlands, New Zealand, Nigeria, Norway, Poland, Saudi Arabia, Slovakia, Slovenia, Sweden, Switzerland (served by Germany), United Kingdom, United States.

The McKenzie Institute holds international conferences every three years, with conferences for the Americas and Europe, respectively, held in the intervening years. At each conference, hundreds of health care professionals gather to learn more about scientific literature as it pertains to conservative management of lower back and extremity pain. Recent international conferences have been held in 2009 (Rio de Janeiro) and 2012 (Austin, Texas). The next will be held in 2015 in Copenhagen. Conferences of the Americas have been presented in Baltimore, Maryland, in 2010 and Denver, Colorado, in 2013. The next will be held in 2016 in a city to be determined.

The McKenzie Institute provides two types of certification for health professionals already licensed by their states, provinces, or nations as physical therapists, chiropractors, or physicians. These are the credentialing certificate and the institute's diploma in Mechanical Diagnosis and Therapy. The certificate entitles the holder to use the term "Cert. M.D.T." (Certificate in Mechanical Diagnosis and Therapy) after his or her name; the diploma permits the use of "Dip. M.D.T." (Diploma in Mechanical Diagnosis and Therapy).

The McKenzie Institute International has established Spinal Therapy and Rehabilitation Centers to provide treatment programs for patients with chronic and recurring back and neck problems, and the institute works directly with referring physicians in formulating ongoing self-treatment programs tailored to the needs of specific individuals.

Further information about the institute's programs is available at the telephone numbers and website noted at the beginning of this appendix.

APPENDIX B
PRODUCTS FOR THE BACK AND NECK

SALES OF THE ORIGINAL MCKENZIE LINE OF LUMBAR AND CERVICAL supports have generated substantial funding for education and research on back and neck pain. Grants have been made in several countries, including the United States, England, and Australia.

PRODUCTS FOR THE BACK

The value of a lumbar roll is discussed in Chapter 4 of this book. The Original McKenzie lumbar roll is constructed of high-quality foam with a durable gray cotton/polyester cover and is available in two densities: regular and firm.

The newest version of the Original McKenzie lumbar roll is the Original McKenzie SuperRoll, which provides long-life lumbar support without significant bulk. You can position the SuperRoll exactly where it is needed and secure it in place with either a hook-and-loop panel or a removable adjusting strap. This product is designed especially for use in automobiles and office chairs.

A wraparound lumbar roll for use when sleeping is also available: the Original McKenzie night roll ties around the waist, presenting an ideal way to help correct the sleeping position as described in Chapter 4 of this book. It is available in three sizes.

PRODUCT FOR THE NECK

Described in Chapter 11 of this book, the Original McKenzie cervical roll supports the neck while you sleep. Designed to slip between your pillow and pillowcase, the cervical roll reduces strain on the cervical discs while providing greater comfort than is available from any pillow alone.

ORDERING INFORMATION:
THE ORIGINAL MCKENZIE ROLLS

The Original McKenzie Rolls described in this book are available in North America from Orthopedic Physical Therapy Products (OPTP) in Minneapolis, Minnesota, USA. For information, including pricing, you may call (612) 553-0452 or write to OPTP, P.O. Box 47009, Minneapolis, MN 55447-0009, USA. Orders may be placed by calling (800) 367-7393 or by visiting www.optp .com. Orders from outside the United States may be made by visiting Spinal Publications New Zealand Ltd. at www.spinalpublications.co.nz or www.the originalmckenzie.com.

ABOUT THE AUTHOR, COLLABORATOR, AND COAUTHORS

ROBIN MCKENZIE

Without embellishment, Robin McKenzie can be called the most prominent physical therapist in the world, the one star in his field. Worldwide, more than twenty thousand health professionals have been trained in McKenzie's methods. Authors praise him. So do the five New Zealand prime ministers who have been his patients. International celebrities who have been treated by McKenzie-trained physical therapists do the same.

A survey of 293 physical therapists completed by researchers at the University of Washington in Seattle concluded that the majority believe Robin McKenzie's approach is the single most useful way to treat back pain.

Robin McKenzie earned honors that set him apart from any other physical therapist in the world.

- In 1982 McKenzie was made an Honorary Life Member of the American Physical Therapy Association "in recognition of distinguished and meritorious service to the art and science of physical therapy and to the welfare of mankind." This association presents only about two honorary life memberships per year.

- In 1983 he was elected a member of the International Society for the Study of the Lumbar Spine. At the time, the society's membership was restricted to 150 members worldwide.
- In 1984 he was elected a Fellow of the American Back Society.
- In 1985 he was awarded an Honorary Fellowship by the New Zealand Society of Physiotherapists.
- In 1987 he was made an Honorary Life Member of the New Zealand Manipulative Therapists Association.
- In 1990 he became an Honorary Fellow of the Chartered Society of Physiotherapists of the United Kingdom.
- In 1990, in the Queen's Birthday Honours, Queen Elizabeth conferred on McKenzie the title Officer of the Most Excellent Order of the British Empire, entitling him to be addressed as "Robin McKenzie, OBE."
- In 1998 he became an Honorary Fellow of the New Zealand College of Physiotherapy.
- In 2000, in the New Year Honours, Queen Elizabeth appointed him to an even higher order, naming him a Companion of the New Zealand Order of Merit (CNZM).

McKenzie wrote four books for health professionals to use with patients being treated for back, neck, shoulder, or knee pain, *Treat Your Own Back*, *Treat Your Own Neck*, *Treat Your Own Shoulder*, and *Treat Your Own Knee*. The books are part of the treatment program for patients. The books have sold a total of more than 6 million copies worldwide. McKenzie also wrote three books for health professionals themselves: *The Lumbar Spine: Mechanical Diagnosis and Therapy*, *The Cervical and Thoracic Spine: Mechanical Diagnosis and Therapy*, and *The Human Extremities: Mechanical Diagnosis and Therapy*. In addition, he wrote *Against the Tide: Back Pain Treatment—the Breakthrough: An Autobiography*. Robin McKenzie died in 2013.

Among those who praise McKenzie are authors of other books on back and neck pain. Judylaine Fine is the founder of the Back Association of Canada, the only charitable foundation in North America devoted to educating back sufferers and those who treat them. She is the author of *Your Guide to Coping with Back Pain*. In that book she writes:

The McKenzie Method approaches disc problems in a totally new way that focuses on soft tissue (mostly muscles and ligaments). . . . But its most revolutionary aspect is the use of extension exercises and the maintenance of the lumbar lordotic curve. . . .

. . . [A]lmost everyone agrees that, for disc problems in particular, extension exercises should be part of the treatment. The fact that our current definition of good posture is dramatically different from what it was just a decade ago has a lot to do with Robin McKenzie.

In 1983, Robin McKenzie became the first physical therapist to be elected to the membership of the prestigious Society for the Study of the Lumbar Spine. To many people, myself included, it felt as if the entire profession was being knighted, not just the man himself. . . . Physical therapists would never use the term, but I can say it: Robin McKenzie was the profession's first star.

COLLABORATOR

Craig Kubey

Craig Kubey is a member of the bars of California and the District of Columbia. As a public interest attorney, he was a cofounder of the Equal Justice Foundation, a national public interest organization in Washington, D.C., established to improve access to justice in courts and regulatory agencies for "average" Americans. After switching careers to writing, Kubey has published nine books, three of them national bestsellers (on the *New York Times*, Amazon. com, or other major lists). Reviewers have called three of Kubey's books the best ever published on their subject. Among Kubey's books are *Pat Summerall's Sports in America* (HarperCollins, a book on thirty-two sports legends, a collaboration with the late sportscaster Pat Summerall), *You Don't Always Need a Lawyer* (Consumer Reports Books, a book on alternatives to lawsuits), *The Viet Vet Survival Guide* (Ballantine Books, a collaborative book instructing American military veterans on how to get VA and other government benefits, even if the government has unfairly denied their claims); he later published an additional collaborative book for vets and a collaborative e-book for vets and current servicemembers, including vets and "SMs" from the wars in Iraq and Afghanistan, and *The Winners' Book of Video Games* (Warner Books, a book on game strategy and the industry). Kubey has benefited dramatically from Robin McKenzie's exercises for both the back and the neck.

COAUTHORS OF THE SHOULDER SECTION

Grant Watson

Grant Watson is a physiotherapist in private practice in Richmond, Nelson, New Zealand. He is a senior international instructor and assistant director for the McKenzie Institute International and has taught extensively in Great Britain, Europe, North and South America, and the Asia Pacific region. He has been actively involved with education within physiotherapy since 1985 and regularly coordinates workshops and publishes articles promoting aspects of self-management, in both the spine and the extremities. He is an accredited physiotherapist to the New Zealand Academy of Sport.

Robert Lindsay

Robert Lindsay is a physiotherapist in private practice in Coromandel Peninsula, New Zealand, with postgraduate qualifications in orthopedic and manipulative physiotherapy. He firmly believes in the role of education and self-treatment within the scope of physiotherapy, as people generally are able to successfully treat and prevent or limit recurrence of many of the soft tissue disorders that occur in daily life.

INDEX

Note: Page numbers in *italics* indicate photographs and illustrations.

accidents, 117, 176, *187, 191*
acromioclavicular (AC) joint,
　183, *183*
acupuncture, 108
acute back pain
　and bed rest, 108
　bulging discs, 20
　and development of McKenzie
　　Method, 6–7
　exercises for, 62–63, 62–65,
　　67, 69, 74, 82–83, 89, 90–94
　immediate self-treatment of,
　　90–94
　medicines and drugs for, 107
　and pain after activity, 103
　in those over 50, 103–4
　treatment precautions, 166
　typical experiences with, 78
acute neck pain
　exercises for, 143, 144, 147,
　　148, 151, 155, 161, 163–64

instructions for, 163–65
　and timing of exercises,
　　158–59, 158–65, 160
　treatment precautions, 169
acute shoulder pain, 141,
　223–27
Agency for Health Care Policy
　and Research, 7, 79
airline seating, 41, 109
American Academy of
　Orthopaedic Surgeons, 172
anatomy, 11–13, 17
annulus (annular ligament),
　12, 113
arthritis, 5, 104, 123, 172
athletes, 99–103. *See also*
　contact sports
automobile accidents, 117

Back Association of
　Canada, 239

Back Exercise 1, Lying
　Facedown, 63–64, *64,* 79,
　80, 81, 86, 89, *93, 167*
Back Exercise 2, Lying Facedown
　in Extension, 63, 64–65, *65,*
　79, 81, 87, 89, *167*
Back Exercise 3, Extension in
　Lying
　case histories, 36, 41, 46–47,
　　51, 57
　described, 66–69, *68,* 76–77
　and frequency/timing of
　　exercises, 73–74, 79, 81, *83,*
　　83–84, 87–88, 89
　and pain after activity, 99, 102
　and pregnancy, 98, 99
　and REPEX treatments, 95
　and self-treatment of back
　　pain, 92
　and sudden acute pain, *167,* 168
　in those over 50, 104

Back Exercise 4, Extension in
    Standing, 41, 46–47, 66,
    69–70, 81, 84, 89, 99, 102
Back Exercise 5, Flexion in
    Lying, 36, 47, 51, 66, 71–74,
    72, 82, 82, 83, 98, 98,
    98–99, 104
Back Exercise 6, Flexion in
    Sitting, 74–76, 75, 98, 98
Back Exercise 7, Flexion in
    Standing, 36, 51, 57, 70, 76,
    76–77, 83, 84, 84
back pain
    anatomy of, 11–13
    economic impact of, 3–4
    guidelines and precautions,
        166–68
    and mechanical pain, 15,
        18–22
    and poor posture, 2–3
    problems described, 2–6
    products for, 235–36
    sudden onset, 166–68
bed rest, 79, 81, 108, 164, 167–68
beds. See lying down position;
    sleeping position
bending, 42. See also slouching;
    stooped working positions
bipedal motion, 13
buttocks, 21

capsulitis, 172, 207
cardiac problems, 176
car seats, 16, 34, 34, 38, 39,
    91–92, 102, 108–10, 174, 174
cartilage, 12
centralization of pain
    case histories, 57, 74
    and frequency/timing of
        exercises, 81, 83, 159
    and the McKenzie Method,
        56–57, 60, 67

and neck pain, 139, 139–40,
    148, 152, 154, 159, 164
cervical collars, 164
cervical lordosis, 30, 116, 117
cervical rolls, 16–17, 38, 133–35,
    134, 135, 164, 236
cervical spine, 16, 113–16
chairs, 16, 33, 92. See also car
    seats
childbirth, 97
chiropractors, 144, 175
chronic back pain
    consequences of, 3
    described, 4–5
    exercises for, 62–63, 65, 78
    lower back pain, 26
    and the McKenzie Institute
        International, 233
    in those over 50, 103–4
chronic neck pain, 233
chronic shoulder pain, 189
clavicle, 116, 183, 183
contact sports, 19, 61, 117, 141
continuous passive motion
    (CPM), 96
coughing, 54

degenerative disc disease,
    5, 66, 104
desk work, 30, 32–33, 132, 157
discs
    anatomy of, 12, 12, 115
    bulging discs, 17, 20, 118
    herniated discs, 98–99
    and neck pain, 113, 118, 132
    and prolonged sitting,
        31, 41
    slipped discs, 5, 111
    and stooped working
        positions, 42
dizziness, 141
driving. See car seats

elastic cartilage, 12
environmental causes of pain,
    32–34, 125–27, 197–200,
    206–7
extension
    described, 6–7, 55
    Mayo Clinic exercises, 137
    and McKenzie Method back
        exercises, 56, 64–65, 65,
        66–69, 68, 69–70, 70
    and mechanical pain,
        14–17, 15
    and osteoporosis, 105–6
    and shoulder pain, 179,
        179–81
    See also specific exercises

falls, 187, 191
fatigue, 95
fibrocartilage, 12
fibromyalgia, 5
fibrositis, 5, 111
Fine, Judylaine, 239
first-aid exercises, 63, 65
flexibility, 82, 115–16, 160,
    194, 227
flexion
    described, 6–7, 55
    extension contrasted with, 17
    and lower back pain, 74
    and McKenzie Method back
        exercises, 56, 71–73, 72,
        74–76, 75, 76
    for stiffness in the back, 73
    See also specific exercises
frozen shoulder, 172, 207, 207–8,
    227, 229–30
furniture design
    and causes of back pain, 32,
        32–34, 108–10, 125–27
    and mechanical pain, 15
    and neck pain, 127

and self-treatment of back
pain, 91
See also car seats

headaches, 155, 157, 161–62
heart problems, 176
herniated discs, 98–99
hip position, 84–88
humerus, 183, *183*, 184

ibuprofen, 79
impingement syndrome, 172
increasing pain, 67, 140
inflammation, 189
intensity of pain, 58–62,
210–11
International Society for the
Study of the Lumbar
Spine, 62
Isometric Abduction in
Standing, Shoulder Exercise
6, 220–21, *221*, 224, 227,
227, 228, 229

*Journal of the American Medical
Association,* 3

Kubey, Craig, 239–40

lifting, 26, *28,* 42–47, *43, 44,* 91,
185, *185,* 190
ligaments, 15
and mechanical pain, 19
and neck pain, 117, 118
and shoulder pain, 190
and sitting for prolonged
periods, 124
and spinal anatomy, 12–13
and stooped working
positions, 42
Lindsay, Robert, 240
location of pain

intensity and movement of
pain, 58–62, 121
localization of pain, 59, 139
lower back pain, 21–23, *22*
and neck pain, 121–22, *122*
and shoulder pain, 177–78,
178, 210–11
and timing of exercises,
159–60
lordosis
after athletic exertion, 102
and causes of back pain, 26
coughing and sneezing, 54
described, 10, *10*
and frequency/timing of
exercises, 81, 82
and furniture design, 32
and lifting technique, 46–47
loss of, 14
and lying down position, 52
and mechanical pain, 16, 18
and neck pain, 116
and pregnancy, 97, *97*
and recurring pain, 89
and self-treatment of back
pain, 90–91
and sitting, 30–33, 35–38, *37,*
40, *204,* 204–5, *205*
and standing, 29, 48–49
See also cervical lordosis;
lumbar lordosis
lower back pain
and athletes, 99–103
exercises for, 62–63, 83
lifting, 42–47
and lumbar rolls, 37–40
and lying down position,
49–51, *50*
and the McKenzie Method, 62
and pregnancy, 96–98
prevalence of, 5
and recurring pain, 88–89

and sites of pain, *22*
and sitting for prolonged
periods, 128
and stooped working
positions, 42
lumbar discs, 31, 41
lumbar lordosis, *10,* 74, 91,
116, 128
lumbar radiculitis, 36, 51
lumbar rolls
case histories, 36, 46, 66, 73, 99
and furniture design, 16, *38, 39*
and lower back pain, 51
and lying down position,
52–53, *53*
and neck pain, 133
and neck posture, 128,
128, 129
and office furniture, *130*
and pregnancy, 98, 99
and prevention, 84
and prolonged sitting, *204,*
204–5, *205*
and self-treatment of back
pain, 91, 92
and significant pain, 79
and sitting posture, 37–40,
38, 39, 40, 102, *102,* 132
and sleeping position, 92,
167–68
sources for, 235–36
and sudden onset neck
pain, 171
and vigorous activity, 48
lumbar spine
and furniture design, 16
and lordosis, 10
and lower back pain, 26
and mechanical pain, 18
and neck pain, 126
and spinal anatomy, *11,* 13
and upright posture, 13

lying down position, 49–53, *50*, 79, *120*, 132–36, 197, *198*, 206. *See also* sleeping position

Mayo Clinic exercises, 105–6, *106*, 137
McKenzie, Robin, 237–39
McKenzie Institute International, 8, 34, 53, 176, 231–33
McKenzie Method
 audience for, 23–25
 and centralization of pain, *60*
 end extension, 6–7
 frequency and timing of exercises, 62, 78–89
 locating credentialed therapists, 231–33
 and new pains, 61
 origin of, 1–2
 research supporting, 62–63
Mechanical Diagnosis and Therapy, 176
mechanical pain, 14–17, 18–22, 116–19, 185–86
medicines and drugs for pain, 79, 107
menopause, 105
midline pain, 83
muscle strain, 18–19, 189

Neck Exercise 1, Head Retraction in Sitting, 126, 129–33, 137, 141–45, 151–52, 154–55, 158–62, 171
Neck Exercise 2, Neck Extension in Sitting, 126, 144–47, 154, 158, 171
Neck Exercise 3, Head Retraction in Lying, 144, 147–49, *148*, 151, 159, *170*

Neck Exercise 4, Neck Extension in Lying, *149*, 149–51, *150*, 159, 162, *170*
Neck Exercise 5, Side Bending of the Neck, 151–52, *152*, 154, 159, *170*, *180*
Neck Exercise 6, Neck Rotation, 152–54, *153*, *155*, 160–61, *180*
Neck Exercise 7, Neck Flexion in Sitting, 137, 155–57, *156*, 162
neck pain
 causes of, 116–19, 124–37
 and cervical spine, 113–14, 115–16
 described, 2–6, 111–13
 guidelines and precautions, 138–42
 and lying down position, *50*
 and mechanical pain, 15
 and posture, 2–3, 116, *117*, *119*, 119–20
 products for, 236
 and self-treatment, 123
 sites of, 121–22, *122*
 and sitting for prolonged periods, 124–32
 sudden onset, 169–71
 timing of exercises, 158–65
neuritis and neuralgia, 111
nonsteroidal anti-inflammatory drugs (NSAIDs), 79, 107
nucleus pulposus, 12, 20, 98–99, 113
numbness and tingling sensations, 51, 121, 148, 176, 177

occupational causes of pain, *173*, 173–74, *174*
office furniture, 15–16, 31, 32, 38, *38*, 126, *130*

Original McKenzie spinal supports, 134–35, 205, 235–36
osteoporosis, 105–6, 137
overpressure, 138, 144
overstretching
 awkward and cramped work positions, 137
 and mechanical pain, 19
 and neck pain, 117, 118
 and shoulder pain, 185–86, *188*, *191*, 192, *199*, *203*
 and sitting for prolonged periods, 124
over-the-counter medications, 79, 107

peripheralization of pain, 59–61, 118, 148, 166, *178*
physical education, 109–10
physical therapy, 113
pillows, 133–35, *134*, 151, 163–64, 206
posture
 and back pain in pregnancy, 97, *97*
 and causes of back pain, 9–10, 29–30
 correcting lying posture, 135–36
 and furniture design, 15–17, *38*, *39*
 and mechanical pain, 19
 and neck pain, 116, 117–18, *119*, 119–20, 138–39, 157, 164–65
 neck posture, *128*, *129*
 and origins of pain, 2–3
 and physical education, 109–10
 prolonged sitting, 30–41

and self-treatment of back
pain, 91
and shoulder pain, 174, 186,
192–94, *193–94*
and sitting for prolonged
periods, 124–25, *125*
and timing of exercises, 104,
161, 162
visible effects of, 30
See also sitting position;
sleeping position; standing
position
pregnancy, 69, 96–98
prevention
and lower back pain, 69
and neck pain, 154
and shoulder pain, 206–7,
228–29
and timing of exercises,
84–85, 161
vs. treatment, 144–47
push-up exercise, 95. *See also*
Back Exercise 3, Extension
in Lying

quadrupedal motion, 13
quality of life, 173

range of motion, 227. *See also*
flexibility
recurring pain, 6, 88–89,
161, 230
relaxation after activity, 47–48,
95, 136, *136*. *See also* lying
down position; sleeping
position
repeated end-range passive
exercise (REPEX), 95–96
rest and recovery, 140, 202–3,
224–27. *See also* bed rest;
lying down position;
sleeping position

retraction, *179*, 179–81. *See also*
specific exercises
rheumatism, 5, 111
rotator cuff, 172, 183–84, *184*,
189, 190, 192, 227
running, 103–4

sacral vertebrae, *11*
sacrum, 18
scapula, 116, 133, 183, *183*, 205
scar tissue, 21, 118
sciatica, 2, 5, 20, 51, 73
self-treatment, 4–5, 7, 90–94,
93, 112, 123, 175–77
Shoulder Elevation in Lying,
Shoulder Exercise 4,
218–19, *219*, 226, *226*
Shoulder Elevation in Standing,
Shoulder Exercise 5,
219–20, *220*, 226, *226*, *228*
Shoulder Extension in Standing,
Shoulder Exercise 2,
214–16, *215*, *216*, 223, *223*,
224, 230
shoulder girdle, 183, *183*,
184, 196
Shoulder Internal Rotation in
Standing, Shoulder Exercise
3, *217*, 217–18, *218*, 225,
225, 228, *228*
shoulder pain
causes, 172–82
chronic, 3
described, 172–75
diagnosing problem, 177–81
and environmental factors,
197–200
exercises for, 209–11, 212–21,
222–30
and frozen shoulder, 207–8
and functions of the shoulder,
184–85

and mechanical pain, 185–86,
186–89
and posture, 173, 192–94,
195–97
prevention of, 206–7
problems described, 2–6
and prolonged sitting/
standing, 203–5
and raised arm postures, *173*,
174, 186, *188*, *191*, *193–94*,
195, *199*, 200–203, *202*
self-treatment of, 175–77,
181–82
and shoulder anatomy,
183–84, 190
and sleeping position, 206
and tissue damage, 189
Shoulder Pendular Exercise,
Shoulder Exercise 1, *213*,
213–14, *214*, 222, 230
Shoulder Strengthening,
Shoulder Exercise 6,
220–21, *221*, 224, 227, *227*,
228, 229
sitting position
and car seats, 16, 34, *34*, 38, *39*,
91–92, 102, 108–10, 174, *174*
and flexion exercises,
74–76, *75*
and furniture design,
38, *39*, *40*
and lumbar rolls, *38*, *39*
prolonged sitting, 30–41,
124–32, 203–5
and self-treatment of back
pain, 91
and shoulder pain,
195–96, *201*
slouching, *27*, *32*
sleeping position
and causes of back pain,
49–51, *50*

sleeping position (*cont.*)
  correcting lying surfaces,
    133–35
  facedown position, *135,*
    135–36, 164
  and neck pain, *120,* 132–36,
    163–64
  and self-treatment of back
    pain, 91
  and shoulder pain, 174, *174,*
    197, *198,* 206
  See also lying down position
slipped disc, 5, 111
slouching
  after vigorous activity, 47–48,
    100–101, *101*
  and frequency/timing of
    exercises, 81
  and mechanical pain, 19
  and neck pain, 126, 129, 133
  and prolonged sitting, 30–31,
    33, 35, *35,* 35–37, 38–39
  and shoulder pain, 193,
    196, *196*
  slouch-overcorrect procedure,
    35–37, 81–82, 126, 133

sneezing, 54
soft tissues, 117, 160, 189
Spinal Therapy and
    Rehabilitation Centers, 233
spine
  after athletic exertion,
    100–101, *101*
  after vigorous activity, 48
  anatomy of, 1–2, *11,* 11–13,
    114, 115
  and location of pain, 59, 61
  and lordosis, 10
  and lower back pain, 18–19
  and seating design, 41
  spinal adjustment, 4
  spinal joints, 136
  spinal manipulation, 4
  and upright posture, 13, 56
  See also cervical spine;
    lumbar spine
spondylosis, 111
sports, 61, 136, *136*
standing position
  correcting, 49, *49*
  and flexion exercises, *76,*
    76–77

poor postures, *28*
and pregnancy, 97–98
prolonged standing, 48–49
and shoulder pain, 195–96
and spinal anatomy, 13, 56
stiffness, 73, 138, 155, 160,
    209, 227
stooped working positions, *42,*
    42–43, *43,* 73

tendons, 172, 184, 189, 190, 227
thoracic vertebrae, *11,* 105
Toyota Motor Corporation, 34

upper back pain, 175
upright posture, 197

vacuuming, 42, 91
vertebrae, 1–2, *12, 115*

walking, 13, 26, 31, 41, 124
Watson, Grant, 240
workplace injuries, 41

*Your Guide to Coping with Back
    Pain* (Fine), 239